FINDING A *Lump*
IN YOUR BREAST

WHERE TO GO ... WHAT TO DO

JUDY C. KNEECE, RN, OCN
BREAST HEALTH SPECIALIST

Fully Revised Edition: 2003; First Edition: 1996
ISBN 1-886665-04-4
Library of Congress Card Number: 95-83276
Printed in the United States of America
Published by EduCare Inc.

To order additional copies of this book, contact:

EduCare Publishing
211 Medical Circle
West Columbia, SC 29169
Phone: 803-796-6100
Fax: 803-796-4150
Internet: www.educareinc.com

Publisher's Cataloging In Publication

Kneece, Judy C.
  Finding a lump in your breast: where to go ... what to do /
 Judy C. Kneece
    p. cm.
Includes bibliographical references and index
    LCCN: 95-83276
    ISBN: 1-886665-04-4

  1. Breast--Examination. 2. Breast--Diseases. 3. Breast--
Cancer. I. Title.

RG493.K64 2003   611'.49
                                  QBI95-20800

TABLE OF CONTENTS

Chapter 5
Nipple Discharge   41

Chapter 6
Common Benign Breast Problems   47

Chapter 7
What Your Healthcare Provider Needs To Know   59

ACKNOWLEDGMENTS

John Coscia, M.D., Radiologist, Executive Director
The Comprehensive Breast Center
Don and Sybil Harrington Cancer Center, Amarillo, Texas

Edward P. Dalton, M.D., F.A.C.S., Breast Surgeon
Immediate Past President National Consortium of Breast Centers
Director, Elliot Hospital Breast Center
Manchester New Hampshire

Cheryl Martin, MSN, APRN, OCN
Director of Nursing, Winship Cancer Institute at Emory
Atlanta, Georgia

Dr. Henry Pennypacker and **Dr. Mark Goldstein**
MammaTech Corporation, Gainesville, Florida

Ervin B. Shaw, M.D., Pathologist
Director of Anatomic Pathology, Lexington Medical Center
West Columbia, South Carolina

Davis Hook, R.Ph.
Hawthorne Pharmacy, Columbia, South Carolina

Richard Santen, M.D.
University of Virginia Charlottesville, VA

Paula Correa, M.A.
The Hormone Foundation, Chevy Chase, MD

**University of South Carolina School of Pharmacy
Drug Information Center**

Debra Strange
Illustrations

Rick Smoak
Photography

ABOUT THE AUTHOR

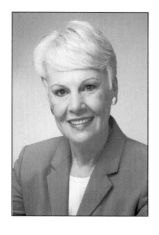

Judy C. Kneece, RN, OCN, is a certified oncology nurse with a specialty in breast cancer and is a MammaCare® Specialist, as well as an author, trainer, and consultant. She presently serves as a national Breast Health Consultant for hospitals and breast centers on the educational and psychosocial needs of the breast patient. She conducts strategic planning and oversees implementation of a comprehensive program of education and support for patients, and trains nurses in a forty-hour training course to fill the role of breast health educator.

Her background as a Breast Health Specialist has allowed her to train thousands of women in breast self-exam skills. It was through this experience that she recognized that women need information about normal and abnormal changes in their breasts and how they can work as a partner with their healthcare providers in monitoring their breast health between clinical exams. She also recognized the need for information by women who have found something suspicious in their breasts, are waiting for an evaluation, or who have high anxiety over monitoring their breasts. To fill this need, she has written this book.

Judy is the author of five books, 35 national journal articles, 291 Patient Education Teaching Topics, *The Breast Health Specialists Manual* and *The Breast Center Strategic Planning Guide*. Her books, *Your Breast Cancer Treatment Handbook, Helping Your Mate Face Breast Cancer* and *Finding a Lump In Your Breast*, have all received outstanding reviews in the Journal of the National Cancer Institute. She is also the author of *Solving the Mystery of Breast Pain* and *Solving the Mystery of Breast Discharge*. She is a contributing editor to major women's magazine articles about breast health, including *Redbook, Marie Claire, Self, Good Housekeeping, Women's Day* and others.

EduCare's Internet site (www.educareinc.com) launched in 1995, was one of the first breast health sites on the web and presently serves approximately 200,000 people per month.

Judy has led efforts in the past several years to research the topics of recurrent breast cancer and its psychological and social impact, and most recently, sexuality issues after chemotherapy. To gather the information, focus groups of survivors were convened across the nation. Data from these focus groups was collected utilizing interactive computers. The final studies have detailed the experience of these survivors and identified their needs for education and support.

As an instructor, Judy has trained and certified over 900 nurses internationally in a forty-hour training course on how to implement programs of education and support for breast health patients in breast centers. In the last ten years she has led an international effort to change the care-delivery of breast cancer patients by (1) identifying breast cancer patient's needs through focus groups, interviews and surveys; (2) instructing nurses on how to deliver patient-focused care in a forty-hour breast health specialist certification program; and (3) leading strategic planning workshops for hospitals to teach how to implement a comprehensive breast care program that includes the psychosocial needs of women.

Judy served as a member of the National Consortium of Breast Centers board of directors for eight years and as the editor of its newsletter, the *Breast Center Bulletin*. She recently served as a guest expert for the American Cancer Society's planning and taping of a new recurrent video series. She presently serves as a member of the Department of Defense Breast Health Scientific Advisory Board representing the interests of breast health patients in the area of educational and psychosocial needs.

As a regular conference speaker and trainer, Judy is best known for her advocacy of the breast cancer patient's psychological and social needs.

DEDICATION

This book is dedicated to all the women who have shared openly their feelings of anxiety after finding a lump in their breasts, having a suspicious mammogram, living as "high risk," or having difficulty with breast self-exam. They served as my motivation to develop materials to help women understand what they need to know and what steps they need to take to protect their health.

I wish to also recognize all of the breast health educators I have trained who take the message of early detection to women by training and teaching them to monitor their breasts.

My gratefulness is extended to, Dee Lucas, Melanie Kneece, Marilyn Dooley, and Dr. Tom Smith for their support in preparing this manuscript.

The best defense against breast cancer is an informed woman, familiar with her own breasts, who recognizes a change that needs evaluation by a healthcare provider and follows recommended surveillance guidelines for clinical exams and mammograms. This book will provide you the information you need to be an active participant in protecting your own breast health.

INTRODUCTION

Finding a lump in your breast, having discharge from a breast, or receiving a "suspicious" mammography report can be the most frightening of all experiences for women. Most women immediately think of cancer. Studies show that 50 percent of all women at some time in their lives will experience either finding a lump themselves or having a mammography report that produces a questionable finding. If this happens to you, know that you are not alone in the experience. The good news is that 80 percent of all suspicious findings biopsied reveal a benign change that is **not** cancer.

What do you need to do when you find a lump or a change in your breast? What do you need to know after a questionable mammography report that says there is something suspicious in your breast? What about lumpy breasts that are difficult to examine? What about painful breasts? What do you do if you have a nipple discharge? Have you been told you have "fibrocystic disease" or are "high risk" and are not sure what this means? Have you had breast cancer surgery and need to monitor your breast(s)? This book is designed to help you understand what to do, where to go and what you need if you have a breast problem. The goal is to help you acquire a healthy knowledge of your breasts, understand common conditions that may occur in your breasts, understand how a healthcare provider may diagnose your problem as well as the latest diagnostic techniques, and learn how you can best work as a partner with your healthcare provider in monitoring your breasts. Understanding your breasts and how to monitor them is an important part of your good health so that abnormal changes can be detected and promptly reported to a healthcare provider. More importantly, you will save yourself needless worry and costly expenses on diagnostic tests that may not be necessary.

Most women know the common, identified risk factors for breast cancer: early menstruation, a history of no children, first child born after age 30, menopause occurring after age 50, or a family history of breast cancer. Diet and the use of hormones have also been suggested as risk factors but have not been consistently proven in studies. An estimated 76 percent of women diagnosed with breast cancer last year had none of the identified risk factors.

The facts are: **no one really knows what causes breast cancer** or who will have breast cancer. The most common risk factor is being female; all women are at risk. All women need to know how to monitor their breast health.

Often women who have identified risk factors are overly anxious about their breast health, and women who think they have no risk factors may neglect their breast health. Being considered "high risk" or experiencing a noncancerous problem may be a blessing because of the increased awareness and compliance to screening recommendations that can result in an early detection of cancer. At the present time, early detection is the best weapon available to win the war against breast cancer. The greatest enemy is late detection. Cancer found early can usually be treated successfully. In fact, cancer localized to the breast has never taken the life of any woman. The cancer has to leave the breast (metastasize) and move to a major organ to become life threatening. So, the major goal in breast care is finding the change early while it is still localized in the breast and is most easily treatable. To accomplish this task takes a partnership between an informed woman and her healthcare team.

A trained woman is the most valuable tool we have against breast disease. You can work as a partner with your healthcare provider in monitoring your good health. Located in the back of this book are tear-out worksheets to help you in this task. *It's time you placed yourself in trained hands . . . your own!*

Good breast health to you!

Judy

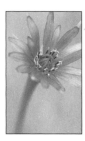

Chapter 1

Why Are My Breasts So Lumpy?

Healthcare providers tell women to check their breasts and notify them immediately if a lump or any change is found. Women often report, however, that when they check their breasts, they are not sure what they are feeling. Often they say their breasts feel very lumpy or ropey and seem to change from one exam to the next. Because of this, many women experience confusion and frustration in managing their breast self-exams. You may have found the same to be true when you checked your breasts. You may also find it hard to know what lumps need to be reported and what is a normal occurrence or change in your breasts.

A breast self-exam becomes easier if you understand how the normal, healthy breast functions. It is estimated that women find 90 percent of all lumps that can be felt in the breast first and then report the finding to their healthcare providers for evaluation. You are the vital link in protecting your breast health. You hold an important key to detection because you can often detect the suspicious change early or between clinical exams by your healthcare provider. As previously stated, early detection is important in breast cancer. The key is a partnership with a healthcare provider by having regular clinical exams, performing breast self-exams regularly, and having mammograms on the schedule your healthcare provider recommends.

Why are my breasts so lumpy? This is the first question to answer so you can understand the normal functioning of your breasts. When you learn what is normal and become familiar with your own pattern of lumpiness, you will then feel more confident in recognizing any change that should be evaluated by a healthcare provider. Let's look at the normal breast.

Understanding Your Breasts

Women can be confused when performing a breast self-exam because they often think that the breast should be soft and spongy. Most expect the tissues to feel like a bowl of Jell-O. In reality, the breasts feel more like a bowl of lumpy oatmeal after it gets cold. This is because the breast is a very complex, glandular (composed of glands) organ that naturally feels lumpy and bumpy.

The breasts lie on the chest wall between the second and sixth ribs. Women with very small breasts may feel their ribs when doing their exam. Strong fibrous tissues that look like a very fine cord, called the Cooper's ligaments, hold the breast to the chest wall. Cooper's ligaments are found throughout the breast and are attached into the pectoralis chest muscle.

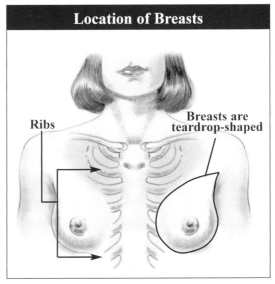

Location of Breasts

Ribs

Breasts are teardrop-shaped

The shape of the breast is much like a teardrop. It is not completely round. The breast extends from what we put into a bra into the area toward our armpit. The glandular (working units under the skin) part of the breast appears much like a daisy, with the nipple in the center surrounded by dark-colored tissue, the areola. The size and color of nipples and areolas (dark circle around nipple) vary in women. The darker the complexion, the darker the areola. Blond women usually have a pinkish-brown areola while those with dark complexions have brownish black areolas. It is common for the areola to turn darker during pregnancy. The nipples protrude above the areola and point slightly toward the armpits. However, some women have naturally inverted nipples that do not protrude. This condition does not affect breast-feeding. Around the areola are also a few hair follicles. It is normal for most women to have some nipple hair. If this bothers you, you can pluck them out, but they are normal. On the areola are oil glands that look like little goose bumps under the skin.

These glands (Montgomery's glands) lubricate the nipple during nursing, but can become infected at any time, just like the oil glands on our face causing a bump or pimple.

Under the skin, the breast gland radiates into 15 to 20 lobes, like the petals of a daisy. Its structure is much like a limb on a tree that has small branches with leaves along the each branch. Beyond the milk ducts, the lobes branch into 20 to 40 lobules. At the end of each lobule are the acini (also called alveoli) where the milk or breast fluid is produced. These small milk-producing units vary in number from 10 to 100 per lobule, according to the amount of hormonal stimulation from estrogen and progesterone.

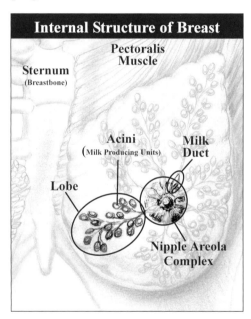

Internal Structure of Breast

Sternum (Breastbone)

Pectoralis Muscle

Acini (Milk Producing Units)

Milk Duct

Lobe

Nipple Areola Complex

Near the nipples the ducts (branches) enlarge into milk ducts (lactiferous sinus) that act as holding tanks for breast fluid. These ducts terminate into an estimated 6 to 10 openings on each nipple. Through these nipple openings comes milk from the ducts, lobes and lobules to which they are connected. They are not connected with other lobe or lobule complexes, which means that if one duct complex becomes diseased, it will drain from only one opening on the nipple and not involve any others. This will be important when we study different signs of disease.

Between all of these glandular parts are fat tissue (it is estimated that 1/3 of the size of breast comes from fat), nerves, lymphatic vessels, blood vessels and lymph nodes, all of which lie under the skin and over the muscles and ribs of the chest wall. You can now understand why you might be confused about what you feel when you perform your breast self-exam. This is why your breasts feel so lumpy.

Why Do My Breasts Feel Different at Different Times?

As you can see from the illustrations, the breast is a very complex organ. To complicate your exam even more, the breast glands have the ability to change in size during the month because ducts increase in cells and the milk-producing glands (acini or alveoli) proliferate. This occurs each month when the female hormones stimulate the breasts to prepare for pregnancy by increasing the number of milk-producing cells and by producing and storing

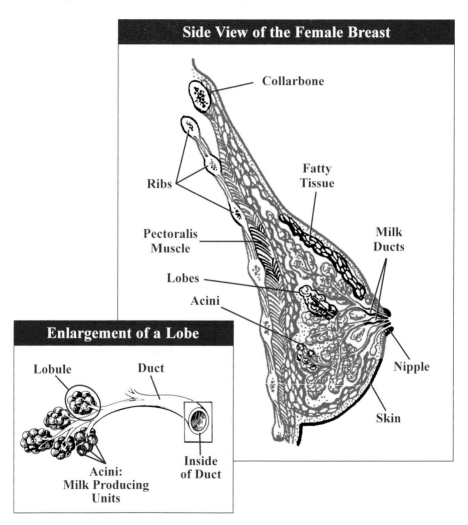

Side View of the Female Breast

Collarbone

Ribs

Fatty Tissue

Pectoralis Muscle

Milk Ducts

Lobes

Acini

Nipple

Skin

Enlargement of a Lobe

Lobule

Duct

Acini: Milk Producing Units

Inside of Duct

breast fluid. Before your menstrual period, the amount of stored fluid in each breast varies from 15 to 30 ccs (three to six teaspoons). This increased fluid retention causes enlargement of the breasts and may cause tenderness or pain. If pregnancy does not occur, the breast has to reabsorb this fluid through the lymphatic system, which picks it up and carries it away.

This gradual growth and filling with fluid of the breast before a menstrual period is the reason the breasts feel different at different times of the month. This is also the reason you may become confused if you randomly examine your breast during different times of the monthly cycle. To prevent such confusion, it is helpful to perform your breast self-exam at the same time in each cycle, preferably when the breasts are least filled with fluid. The least amount of fluid retention is seen in the week after the menstrual period. However, the goal is not so much finding the day, but rather that you choose the same time in each cycle so that you will become familiar with the amount of engorgement and filling that is normal for you at that time of your menstrual cycle. Checking your breasts the same time in each cycle helps you become the expert on your normal pattern of breast lumpiness. There is no magic about one day, but the secret to becoming an expert on your breasts is that you perform the exam the same time during your cycle.

You want to select a time when your breasts are least tender and not filled with fluid. The best time to check your breasts varies according to the stage in your life:

- **Menstruating women**—the last day of the menstrual period is the easiest time to remember consistently. This serves as your monthly reminder, making it less likely to be forgotten.

- **Menopausal and pregnant women**—the same day each month.

- **Women on hormonal therapy who cycle off for several days**—the day you resume your medication.

- **Breastfeeding mothers**—when all milk has been expressed from the breast (this sometimes means that only one breast can be checked at a time because all the milk cannot usually be expressed completely from both breasts).

For a complete guide to breast self-exam, refer to Chapter 14.

What Is Normal Nodularity?

The breasts will feel very lumpy near the beginning of the monthly period and will be least engorged and lumpy at the end of the menstrual period. The body's normal response to hormones causes the breast to change and feel lumpy during the month and is called **normal nodularity**. Because every woman responds differently and has varying amounts of hormonal stimulation, each woman's breasts are unique in their pattern of lumpiness or texture. Some areas in the breast will feel more nodular. These normal patterns of lumpiness in the breasts are called **patterns of nodularity**.

You need to become familiar with your normal pattern of nodularity. This will allow you to detect an abnormal occurrence—one that is not associated with your normal pattern of hormonal changes during your monthly cycle—if it occurs. Breasts undergo almost daily change, especially during the years from puberty to menopause. The amount of nodularity will also change at different times in your life. The menopausal breast loses most of its glandular tissues, which are replaced with fatty tissues. However, if you take estrogen replacement medications, your breasts may continue to be nodular. It is impossible for a healthcare provider to get to know your breasts and their pattern of normal nodularity as well as you can because the provider examines your breasts only once a year. A self-exam helps you learn your normal patterns of nodularity and recognize any unusual change in them. Therefore, a regularly practiced breast self-exam becomes very important in detecting abnormal changes early.

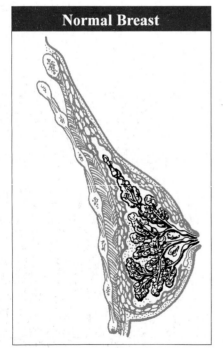

Normal Breast

Normal Breast

The breast is composed of glandular tissue that varies in nodularity (lumpiness, texture) during the month because of hormonal level changes. These monthly changes start at menstruation and continue until menopause.

Pregnant Breast

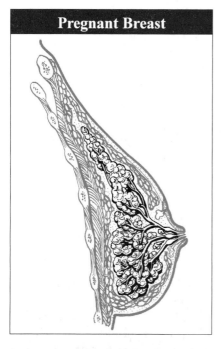

Pregnant Breast

Glandular tissues are stimulated by changes in hormone levels and enlarge. The acini, the milk-producing glands, proliferate and may number as high as 100 at the end of each lobule as they prepare to produce milk during breast-feeding.

Menopausal Breast

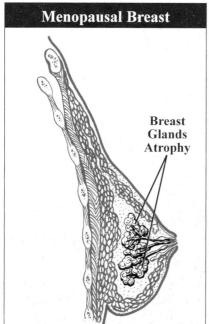

Breast
Glands
Atrophy

Menopausal Breast

The glandular tissue in the breast atrophies—decreases in size. The breast fills with fatty tissues and it feels much softer. The breasts naturally begin to sag after menopause. Breast self-exam becomes much easier and mammography is able to visualize the area more accurately because of the decrease in the dense glandular tissue. Hormonal supplements will decrease the amount of loss of glandular tissue and breast sagging.

How Do You Know If
What You Feel Is Normal Nodularity?

What does normal breast nodularity feel like? The texture of a normal breast is described as a generalized lumpiness with no **firm, obvious, single hard lump**. A feeling of ropiness comes from the strong glandular and fibrous tissues of the breast. An area of the breast may also feel as if there are grains of sand under the skin; this is caused by the increased size of the acini that produce the breast fluid. If you use deep pressure, you may feel the ribs under the breast tissue. Ribs are often mistaken for breast lumps. The area under the nipple will feel distinctly firmer from the converging of the large lactiferous milk glands.

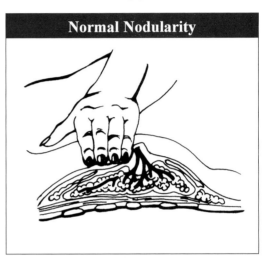

Normal Nodularity

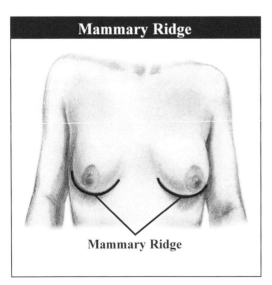

Mammary Ridge

Mammary Ridge

There is an area at the base of the breast (bra underwire area) that has a distinct feeling of thickening; this is called the **mammary ridge** or **inframammary ridge**. This is also a normal finding.

What About The Size of My Breasts?

All female breasts are composed of the same glandular tissues that undergo the same monthly changes due to hormonal response. However, the size of breasts varies among women. Some have very small breasts and some very large. The size of breasts is inherited genetically but can be influenced by hormonal stimulation or weight gain or weight loss. It is estimated that about one third of the size is from fat. The amount of fat in the breast varies as your body fat does. So, the breasts are one of the sites that lose or gain weight as you do. One breast is usually slightly smaller than the other and one may also sit higher on the chest wall.

Size of the breasts has nothing to do with a woman's ability to produce breast milk to feed a baby. Small breasts respond to the hormones of pregnancy just as larger breasts do. Neither does size have anything to do with the risk of having cancer of the breast.

Very large breasts may be uncomfortable physically and cause many physical problems including neck and back pain and present a challenge when buying clothing. Some women find that having breast reduction is the answer for their problem. Small-breasted women may choose to have their breasts enlarged (augmented) with implants or their own body tissue. The ideal size of breast is the size that you feel comfortable with, and we should never be pressured by society to feel there is a perfect size for breasts.

Large breasts also require more time for breast self-exam. The secret for examining large breasts is found in using three levels of pressure when you examine your breast and a side-lying position for the first half of your exam. This technique is described in the new MammaCare® method explained in Chapter 14. There is no increased risk for breast disease in large breasts, only the increased challenge of performing an exam.

Remember:

- The female breast is not a soft spongy organ, but a very complex glandular organ that changes during the monthly cycle and at different stages during a woman's life.

- Becoming familiar with the normal patterns of nodularity of your breasts is your best assurance of recognizing changes early.

Internal Structure of the Breast

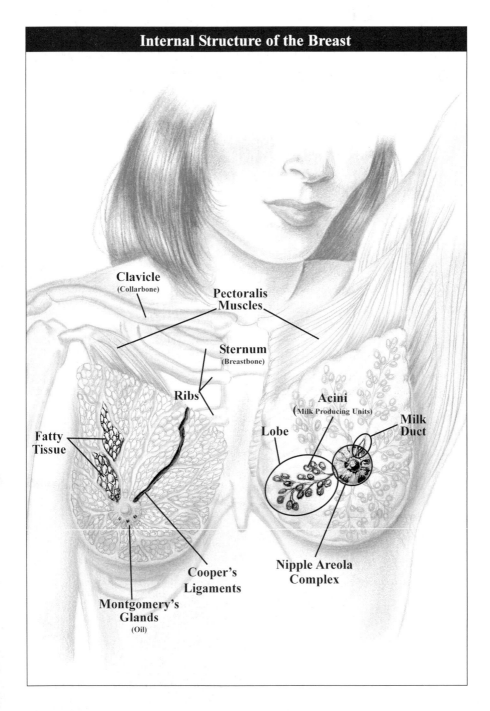

CHAPTER 2

WHEN YOU FIND A CHANGE IN YOUR BREAST

What you will be checking for in your breast self-exam are **changes** from the normal. A change you can feel that needs an evaluation by a healthcare provider is most often a **distinct lump**, a **new area of thickening**, **retraction of the skin or nipple**, a **nipple discharge**, and, least likely, **localized breast pain**.

What should you do if you find a lump or change during your exam?

Follow these suggestions:

- As you feel the change, think very carefully about how the lump feels and where it is located in your breast.

- Check the opposite breast in the same area for a similar occurrence.

- If the opposite breast has a similar feeling, these are probably normal hormonal changes. It is usually safe to wait through your next menstrual period if you find similar changes in both breasts.

- If the area you found becomes smaller or softer after a menstrual cycle, it is probably a normal hormonal change. Continue to monitor the area.

- If the area becomes harder or increases in size after observing through a menstrual period, a healthcare provider should examine the area.

- If the suspicious area is a distinct hard lump with no other similar finding in either breast, **contact your healthcare provider**.

What Does Cancer Feel Like?

How does a cancerous lump usually feel? Most women wonder how they would know a cancerous lump from normal nodularity. The **majority** of breast cancer **usually** has the following characteristics.

- One **very firm lump**—it feels like a hardened pea or bean in your breast.

- **Immobile mass**—it does not move freely in the breast.

- Feels **anchored** in the surrounding tissues—when you move the lump, the tissues around it also move.

- **Painless**, approximately 90 percent of the time.

- **One lump** in **one** breast; very rarely will breast cancer appear with several lumps in one breast or in both breasts simultaneously.

However, it is very important to remember that some cancers are not stone hard and are not anchored to surrounding tissues. They may be firm and move freely in your breast like a breast cyst. For this reason, any singular lump that remains in your breast should be evaluated.

Changes You Can See

Remember, we use the word **usually** when describing signs shown by 90 percent of breast cancers during an exam. Most cancers will have these characteristics, but in 5 to 10 percent of breast cancer cases, the cancer does **not** appear as a hard lump. The cancer may occur in both breasts and may **not** show up on mammography. You can look further for changes with a **visual exam** of the breast. When you perform your self-exam, you will also need to look closely at your breasts using a mirror in bright light. Compare the look of one breast to the other to detect visual differences. Changes you observe in your breasts that need evaluation by a healthcare provider are:

- Nipple discharge or one nipple that has a dry, crusty discharge residue

- Inverted nipple that is not normally inverted

- Change in the normal size or shape of the breast—getting larger or smaller

- Change in the normal size or shape of the areola (pulling out or pulling inward)

- Skin changes— redness, blueness, rash, bump, or sore
- Skin dimpling (retraction)
- Bulge
- Vein pattern change (increase to one breast)

Nipple discharge—a bloody discharge or a spontaneous discharge of any color from **one** breast; a persistent discharge from **both** breasts that does not occur right before a menstrual period or following sexual stimulation of the breasts.

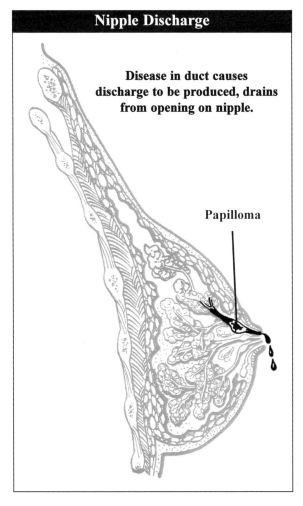

Nipple Discharge

Disease in duct causes discharge to be produced, drains from opening on nipple.

Papilloma

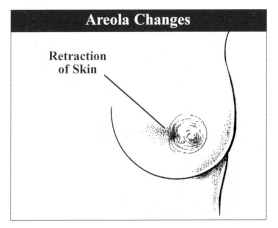

Areola changes—
the pulling out or pulling
in of the circle.

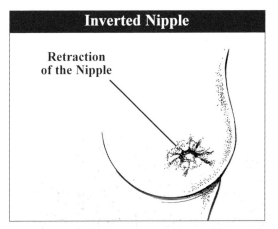

Inverted nipple—
a nipple that inverts in a
previously normal breast.

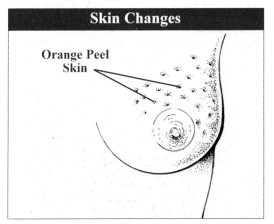

Skin changes—
redness of the breast,
irritation or redness of the
nipple, a bump or sore, or
skin that looks pitted like
an orange peel.

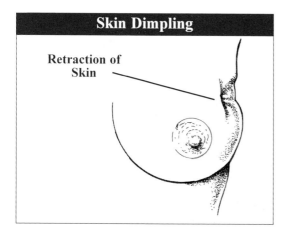

Skin dimpling—
a pulling in of the skin, creating a retraction of the area.

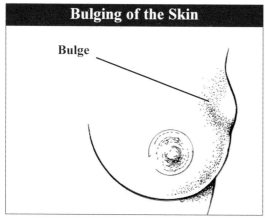

Bulging of the skin—
a protrusion of one area of the breast that creates a change in the shape of the breast.

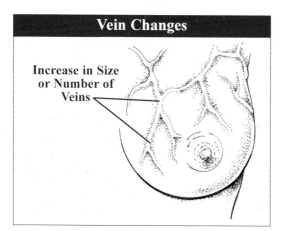

Vein changes—
an increase in the size or number of veins you can see on one breast.

Shape of the breasts—compare the shape of one breast to the other; the shapes should be very similar. Observe the direction in which your nipples point. They should point in similar or symmetrical directions, slightly toward the arm. Most women have one breast that is larger than the other. If one breast begins to decrease or increase in size, this should be reported.

> ## *Remember:*
>
> ■ A visual inspection of your breasts is an important part of monitoring your breast health because some cancers do not form a hard lump. Report any change you may find to a healthcare provider. **A single hard lump always needs evaluation**.

Does Breast Cancer Occur Suddenly?

Contrary to what most people think, the majority of breast cancers do **not** grow rapidly. Breast cancers grow at different rates and double in size (grow from one to two cells, from two to four, then four to eight, etc.) in time spans varying from 23 to as many as 209 days. At an average doubling time of 100 days, most cancers one centimeter large (3/8 inch, the size of the tip of your smallest finger) have been in a woman's body for eight to ten years. Most cancers do not double very rapidly. However, some types of breast cancer found in younger women have very rapid growth patterns. Because you can never be sure of the composition of the lump or change observed, you need to alert a healthcare provider as soon as possible so the area can be monitored.

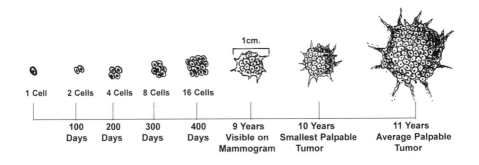

1 Cell	2 Cells	4 Cells	8 Cells	16 Cells	1cm.		
	100 Days	200 Days	300 Days	400 Days	9 Years Visible on Mammogram	10 Years Smallest Palpable Tumor	11 Years Average Palpable Tumor

When You Don't Think You Can Check Your Own Breasts

Some women feel inadequate to attempt examining their own breasts, may be confused by the lumpiness of normal nodularity, or are overwhelmed by the thought that they might find something suspicious. If you feel you would like to become more confident and adept at this skill, call and schedule an appointment with your healthcare provider for a breast exam. It is best to schedule your appointment at the end of your menstrual period.

During the exam, ask the healthcare provider to explain what is being found and to allow you to feel anything that may later confuse you. This allows you to begin your breast self-exam knowing that your breasts have no abnormal lumps at this time and knowing what you will feel is a normal occurrence for you. You will then be able to monitor your breasts for distinct changes.

Hospitals, breast centers and the American Cancer Society often have classes to teach the breast self-exam procedure. Ask your healthcare provider for information about such classes in your area.

Learning how to perform a breast self-exam, including visual inspection of the breasts, enables you to use the most cost-effective and timely method available for early detection. You can monitor your breasts without any costs involved. A majority of lumps large enough to be felt are first found by women rather than their healthcare providers. Many of these are found the months between clinical exams. Training will prepare you to monitor your breasts with more confidence.

Misconceptions About Breast Cancer

People have many misconceptions about breast cancer. Untruths believed by many cause much ill-founded fear. Truths about breast cancer are:

- An injury to the breast does **not** cause breast cancer.

- Sexual stimulation to the breast does **not** cause breast cancer.

- Breastfeeding or mastitis from breastfeeding does **not** cause breast cancer.

- Breastfeeding does **not** prevent breast cancer.

- Breast cancer is **not** transmitted to a nursing child through breast milk.

- Having large breasts or lumpy breasts does **not** increase your risk for breast cancer.

- Having a family history of breast cancer does **not** mean you will have breast cancer.

- Radiation received during mammography does **not** cause breast cancer.

- Antiperspirants are **not** a proven cause of breast cancer.

- Breast cancer is **not** caused mainly by a genetic mutation passed on by parents.

- Women are **not** the only ones to get breast cancer; men can also have it.

- A breast cancer diagnosis is most often **not** a medical emergency.

- Having been told by a healthcare provider you have "fibrocystic disease" does **not** mean you are at a higher risk for breast cancer.

- Breast cancer is **not** contagious.

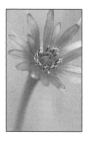

CHAPTER 3

FIBROCYSTIC CHANGES

Most changes and lumps you find in your breast will not be breast cancer. Many changes will be a benign process that will require further evaluation by a healthcare provider. The most common types of benign changes and problems women have in their breasts are discussed briefly in the following chapters.

Fibrocystic Changes

The term "fibrocystic changes or condition," formerly referred to as **fibrocystic disease,** is used to describe a group of changes in the breasts that can be felt and that fluctuate with the menstrual cycle. Changes in hormones during the menstrual cycle cause breast tissues and blood vessels to swell, milk glands and ducts to enlarge, and the breasts to retain water. The uterus, preparing for menstruation, also undergoes changes simultaneously because of the change in the hormonal balance. At this time, the breasts may feel swollen, tender, lumpy, and painful. Some women may form fluid-filled cysts. These changes, which **do not indicate disease**, were previously described as "chronic cystic mastitis" or "mammary dysplasia." The changes are a **normal hormonal response**, common to many women. They are not a sign of a disease.

Some women will have more pronounced symptoms of lumpiness or pain from hormonal changes. Lumpiness and pain are the most frequently occurring breast conditions seen in women. Ninety percent of women have microscopic fibrocystic changes, and 50 percent have changes that can be felt. These changes were once thought to be a pre-condition for breast cancer but are now considered a **normal response** to the monthly hormonal fluctuations of a woman's body.

As the levels of hormones rise and fall, the breast tissues respond by developing some degree of lumpiness. The change is usually associated with pain and tenderness and fluctuates with the menstrual cycle, becoming more noticeable before menstruation. The lumpiness, pain and tenderness stop after menopause, but can recur when hormonal therapy is used for treating menopausal symptoms. Occasionally, with an exaggerated hormonal response, the lumpiness may be difficult to distinguish and a biopsy may be required to determine the exact nature of the lumpiness.

The term **fibrocystic "disease"** has been used by healthcare providers to describe a number of non-cancerous changes in the breast. Many women have experienced much fear and anxiety about their breast health, thinking they have an ongoing disease process in their bodies. If you are told that you have fibrocystic changes, ask your physician exactly what changes have been found.

Many types of treatment are used to ease the symptoms of lumpy, painful breasts, including vitamin supplements, properly fitted bras, hormonal treatments, and restrictions of salt and caffeine (coffee, tea, colas, chocolate). In the following chapter we will discuss how you can tell if your breast pain is related to hormonal changes, medications or other causes, and what you can do to relieve the pain. Caffeine reduction helps many women; however, it may take several weeks or months to evaluate its effectiveness. Refer to Chapter 12 for *The Caffeine Connection*, a guide to amounts of caffeine found in beverages and medications. Chapter 16, *The Drug Connection and Breast Problems*, identifies medications known to cause or exacerbate fibrocystic changes causing breast pain and tenderness.

Remember:

- The term fibrocystic is a term that has been used to describe many changes in the breasts. Ask your physician what is meant if you are told you have fibrocystic "disease." Most often the term refers to changes that are **normal** hormonal changes causing pain and lumpiness, **not an actual disease**.

- The good news is that this diagnosis does not indicate an increased risk for cancer, although it may cause physical discomfort.

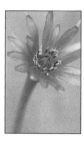

CHAPTER 4

BREAST PAIN

Pain in one or both breasts can cause a woman a lot of anxiety. The majority of breast pain occurrences may be uncomfortable and annoying, but they are usually not unbearable. What seems unbearable is the fear that the pain may be caused by cancer. However, studies show that only a **very small percentage** of breast pain is associated with breast cancer. Almost all breast pain is due to other causes. It is estimated that only approximately 10 percent of breast cancers that are palpable have pain as a symptom. A healthcare provider's careful history, examination, and mammogram can often determine the cause of breast pain. After ruling out cancer, a close investigation of the possible type of pain and pain management needed can be implemented.

Two major types of breast pain have been identified—**cyclic and noncyclic**. Cyclic breast pain corresponds with monthly hormonal changes which sometimes promote pain. Noncyclic breast pain does not correspond with the increase or decrease in hormonal stimulation from your menstrual cycle on the breast tissues.

Cyclic Pain

The most common pain, cyclic pain (often called fibrocystic changes or condition), is related to the female hormones and their monthly effect on the breasts. This pain begins at ovulation and increases until menstruation begins, which relieves the degree of pain. The pattern of occurrence correlates with pre-menstrual syndrome (PMS), increasing in degree as the menstrual period approaches. It is estimated that 60 - 75 percent of all pain is caused by cyclical hormones.

Pain occurs in both breasts with cyclic pain. However, pain may be greater in one breast. Discomfort is most often greatest in the upper, outer breast quadrant (from the nipple back toward the armpit). The pain is described as dull and aching, as if the breasts were filled with milk. They may be tender when touched and feel heavy. Pre-menopausal women experience this pain. Menopause relieves the symptoms of true cyclic breast pain. However, women who take estrogen replacement therapy (ERT) may experience pain when medication is begun. If the pain continues past several months, a healthcare provider should check to see if the level of the medication is too high. Pain should not be a continued occurrence if ERT is prescribed.

Medical literature has attributed cyclic breast pain to increased levels of estrogen in relationship to progesterone. Other studies have shown that elevated levels of the hormone prolactin (a hormone that stimulates milk production) can also be a cause of cyclic pain.

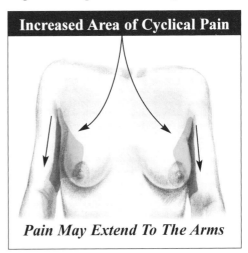

Increased Area of Cyclical Pain

Pain May Extend To The Arms

<u>Noncyclic Pain</u>

Noncyclic pain differs from cyclic pain in that it has no relationship to changing hormone levels and the menstrual cycle. The pain may be continuous, or it may only occur from time to time. The pain is usually localized to a specific area in one breast. It is often described as a sharp stabbing or burning sensation in the breast. Noncyclic pain may be caused by breast disease (benign or malignant), bone or muscle pain (musculoskeletal) or direct injury to the breast.

Breast disease pain has been linked to fluid-filled cysts or fibroadenomas that press on a nerve, duct ectasia, mastitis, injury and breast abscesses. An under-functioning thyroid gland (hypothyroidism) can also cause breast pain. While breast cancer may be the source of pain, it is not common, with only 10 percent of palpable cancers causing breast pain, and this is only a fraction of total breast pain incidence itself. Each of the conditions listed here will be discussed in the following chapters.

Some noncyclic pain is also related to musculoskeletal causes. The most common cause of this pain is a pinched nerve in the back. The pain originates from the nerve located along the spinal column and is referred to the breast, causing it to feel as if the pain is located there. A history of back injury, scoliosis, arthritis, or osteoporosis can all be causes of breast pain. As mentioned previously, usually only one breast will be painful.

Another cause of musculoskeletal breast pain originates in the area of the breastbone and ribs and is known as Tietze's syndrome, or **costochondritis** (inflammation of the cartilage between the ribs). The pain is localized close to the breastbone and the area is tender when pressure is placed on the breastbone, when moving the rib cage, or when taking a deep breath. This pain often occurs after heavy lifting or activities that stretch the upper body. Young mothers often suffer from costochondritis from the lifting of children. Athletes suffer more often than other women do from this type of breast pain. Aspirin or ibuprofen (over-the-counter anti-inflammatory medications) will help this pain considerably. It may require 24 to 48 hours for the medication to reduce the pain. Most women receive relief from pain with anti-inflammatory medications taken on a regular schedule during the period of inflammation and by avoiding the activity that promoted the strain on the rib cage. Occasionally, the pain may require an injection of a steroid into the area to reduce inflammation thus reducing or eliminating the pain.

Common Promoters of Breast Pain

Breast pain has also been linked to some medications. Hormonal, blood pressure, psychiatric, gastrointestinal, antidepressant, and heart medications, along with some herbal products, may cause breast tenderness and pain in some women (refer to Chapter 16).

There has been an increase in reports of breast pain from many of the supplements used to promote weight loss (often called "fat burners") and increase energy. The Food and Drug Administration (FDA) finds that they may contain ingredients that stimulate the body in the same manner as caffeine. Ma Huang (Ephedra Sinica or Chinese Ephedra) is a botanical source of ephedrine, pseudoephedrine, and norpseudoephedrine that is found in many of these weight-loss or energy enhancing products. Guarana or Kola Nut, found in many of these supplements, is in reality a type of caffeine.

Many of the herbal products (especially Ginseng and Dong Quai) recommended for treating pre-menstrual symptoms (PMS) and menopausal symptoms may cause some women to experience an onset of breast pain. A diet high in soybean products (found in many liquid diets) or tofu may also cause some women to have breast tenderness or pain. These products produce an estrogen-like effect on the body.

As with any medication, people respond differently, and some women may be very sensitive to these products. When evaluating the cause of your breast pain, consider the use of any medications or supplements in these categories as being possible promoters.

A poor-fitting bra that allows excessive movement of the breasts may be a cause of pain. Infected teeth can also cause pain that is transmitted to the breasts.

How to Determine Which Type of Pain You Have

As you can see, there are many causes of breast pain. Sometimes it will be easy to identify the cause; other times it may take a period of observing your lifestyle to find the cause. If pain is sudden and severe, chronic, or accompanied with a lump or discharge, it should be evaluated by your healthcare provider. A history of the pain and its characteristics will be the first step of evaluation, followed by a clinical breast exam. A mammogram or ultrasound may be ordered by your healthcare provider for additional evaluation. These steps will help determine if a disease in the breast is causing your pain.

If your pain is not caused by breast disease, you can help your healthcare provider determine which type of pain you are experiencing by keeping a monthly calendar. Mark the time you begin and end your menstrual cycle on the calendar and record any activities, any medication, the amount of caffeine consumed, and the degree of pain that you are experiencing each day. A record of this sort helps determine if the pain is cyclic or noncyclic and what may influence or promote your breast pain. Most pain can be categorized in one or two months with the help of your record keeping. Remember, the majority of pain is not related to cancer but to benign causes, but all pain needs evaluation. Tear-out worksheets to collect your pain history and a calendar to monitor your pain are provided in the back of this book.

Comparison of Cyclic, Noncyclic, and Musculoskeletal Pain

FEATURE	CYCLIC	NONCYCLIC	MUSCULOSKELETAL
Age of Onset	20s-30s	30s-40s	Any Age
Location	Bilateral Upper Outer Area	Unilateral One Area	Near Breastbone Usually One Breast
Area of Breast	Spread Out	One Spot	Different Parts of Breast
Type of Pain	Dull, Aching	Sharp, Stabbing	Burning, Aching
Status	Pre-Menopausal	Pre- or Post-Menopausal	Any Age
Hormone Treatment	Responds Well	Minimal Response	No Response
Ibuprofen or Aspirin	Some Help	Some Help	Very Helpful

Pain Management Remedies

If your healthcare provider finds that your pain is from disease, from bone or muscle sources, or injury, they will initiate the appropriate treatment for the specific cause. After you have explored with your healthcare provider the cause of your pain and found that it is not related to a treatable disease, there are specific remedies you may try. Women report they have found improvement in their breast pain with a variety of interventions. Some recommended are dietary, some are mechanical, and some are prescription drugs.

Dietary Therapies

■ Cyclic pain may respond to a reduction of caffeine and caffeine-containing products in your diet (refer to Chapter 12 for instructions and caffeine-containing product lists). Caffeine is a methylxanthine, a chemical that some women find increases symptoms of fibrocystic changes. Reducing your caffeine intake is a simple change you can make in your diet. But remember, it may take months for an accurate evaluation of the effect caffeine has on your body. One or two week's reduction is not an adequate trial for breast pain.

- Reduction of salt in the diet, especially during the second half of the menstrual cycle, helps reduce fluid retention in the body and breast tissues. Increasing your consumption of water will also help the body eliminate excessive sodium and is a healthy dietary habit.

- Low fat diets can reduce the amount of estrogen your body makes. Because estrogen is a steroid hormone, the body needs fat to produce it. A low-fat diet can reduce the amount of stimulation your breasts receive from your own hormones and possibly help in reducing your breast pain. It is recommended that only 20 to 25 percent of your caloric intake come from fat. Never go on a non-fat diet; this is not healthy. Find a fat gram book and learn to count your fat grams, keeping your grams in the recommended range. Increase your consumption of fresh fruits and vegetables. This is another simple, healthy way to address breast pain causes and possibly find relief.

- Vitamin and mineral supplements have proven helpful to some women. Vitamin E has been shown in some studies to reduce breast pain. Because very high doses of vitamins can also have negative side effects, it is recommended that you check with your healthcare provider on the appropriate dosages.

- Evening Primrose Oil has been reported to reduce pain for some women. Like other dietary changes, it may take several months to fully evaluate the change this fatty acid can provide. This is one of the most effective therapies for breast pain. Pregnant women should not take this or any other supplement without checking with their healthcare providers.

Mechanical Therapies

- A properly fitted support bra that minimizes movement of the breast is effective for many women. Wearing a sports bra when sleeping and exercising may also be helpful. Avoid going braless. A good-fitting bra stabilizes the breasts and prevents stretching of the nerve fibers that can cause pain.

- Large-breasted women should choose bras with wide instead of narrow straps. Narrow bra straps that leave indentations on your shoulder can be a cause of breast pain.

- A heating pad or hot bath or shower is helpful for some women. Others find that an ice pack will ease their pain. Heat or cold may reduce swelling and thus reduce pain.

- Breast massage may also reduce pain by helping to remove excess fluid through the lymphatic system. Put lotion on your hands to reduce friction. Make dime-size round circles over all of the breast tissues just as you do during a breast self-exam. Start at the bra line and make straight lines up to your collarbone. Repeat another row starting at the bra line. This increases the removal of fluid from the breast tissues. Some massage therapists specialize in removing accumulated fluid from the breast tissues.

These methods are all free or inexpensive and have no negative side effects. They work by reducing the stretching or irritation of nerve fibers or by eliminating dietary products that can affect breast tissues. Keep your healthcare provider informed as you explore ways to reduce your pain.

Drug Therapies

- Bromocriptine and Danazol (only FDA approved drug for breast pain) both relieve cyclical breast pain by blocking certain hormones (such as estrogen, progesterone or prolactin). The problem with these drugs is that many women find the side effects troublesome. Bromocriptine side effects include nausea, dizziness, and fertility problems. Side effects of Danazol may include weight gain, amenorrhea (no menstrual periods), acne, and masculinization (unwanted facial hair) when given in doses that reduce pain.

- Progesterone supplementation (not progestin, the synthetic form) has been found by many women to be highly effective in treating breast pain. It is based on the emerging theory that breast pain occurs when estrogen levels are too high and out of balance with progesterone. Progesterone is available over-the-counter as a cream and by prescription as an oral micronized (improves absorption) capsule, drops, lozenges or in vaginal suppositories. Compounding pharmacists can take the natural progesterone and compound it into the most suitable form for you. To locate a compounding pharmacist near you, call 800-927-4227. It is necessary that creams purchased over-the-counter contain bio-identical progesterone, most often made from wild yams that have the diosgenin extracted and converted in a laboratory to bio-identical progesterone.

- Birth control pills may also be prescribed for breast pain. The levels of hormones during the perimenopausal years can become very sporadic, causing estrogen to become very high while levels of progesterone are naturally becoming lower. Birth control pills can cause these levels to become more stable, thus reducing or eliminating breast pain.

- Occasionally, pain that is noncyclical and located in one area of the breast may be treated with an injection of anesthetics or corticosteroids to relieve it if it is chronic. A physician would determine if this is a option after a full evaluation of the breast for the cause of the pain.

- Hypothyroidism (low thyroid function) is also associated with chronic breast pain. The pain occurs in both breasts and does not improve greatly after a menstrual period. Evaluation of thyroid function is warranted and if levels are found to be low, supplementation with thyroid medication is indicated for treatment.

Breast Cancer and Pain

Pain with breast cancer is rare and is usually associated with large tumors or tumors pressing on a nerve. In one large study, less than 10 percent of all cancers that could be felt had any pain involved. Women should be aware that a very aggressive type of breast cancer, inflammatory breast cancer, can cause shooting pain through the breast. Onset is sudden and in one breast. Pain is usually accompanied with rapid changes in the color and texture of the breast, which may or may not itch, and an increase in its size can occur in days or weeks.

Remember:

- Breast pain is most often called cyclic breast pain when caused by an imbalance or change in female hormones.

- Noncyclic breast pain is less common and is caused by benign breast disease or injury, muscle or bone origins, and is occasionally associated with cancer.

- All pain should be evaluated thoroughly by a healthcare provider.

- Interventions to relieve the pain should be implemented until pain is resolved or tolerable.

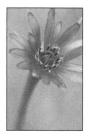

CHAPTER 5

NIPPLE DISCHARGE

Nipple discharge is a common breast complaint with three basic causes:

- Normal hormonal (physiological)
- Medication induced (pharmacological)
- Benign or malignant disease in breast duct

Studies have shown that a normal nipple discharge can be found in 50 to 80 percent of women when no disease is present. Most women have some small amount of discharge when their breasts are squeezed, and this is normal. But **all spontaneous discharge needs to be evaluated** to determine its primary cause.

Normal Discharge

Normal discharge is usually from both breasts (bilateral) and multiple duct openings on the nipple. The appearance of the fluid ranges from opaque to milky (normal color of breast fluid). A woman's natural hormones stimulate production of the discharge. It occurs most often the week before her menstrual period. The breast begins mid-cycle to prepare for potential pregnancy with the proliferation (growth) of the milk-producing acini. During this time fluid is produced and stored in the breast ducts (3 - 6 teaspoons per breast). This explains why the fluid can appear if the breast is squeezed or compressed. If pregnancy does not occur, this fluid is reabsorbed by the body. Sexual stimulation to the breasts can also cause fluid release from the breasts. Excessive squeezing or manipulation can actually encourage the breasts to produce fluid. Stimulation of the breast causes an increase in the production of prolactin, which signals the breast to produce more breast fluid. Aerobic exercises or jogging can cause the breast to bounce up and down on the chest wall and promote a discharge. Women who sleep on their stomach may notice discharge on their nightclothes. Trauma to the breast area and surgery to the chest area can also increase or cause discharge from the breasts.

Women experience an increase in discharge around menopause when the hormones are often sporadically high. In other words, an occasional small amount of discharge from breasts is normal.

A normal discharge has the following characteristics:

- Occurs during the menstrual years, most often the week before the menstrual period

- Occurs in both breasts and comes from multiple duct openings on the nipple

- Looks opaque or milky colored

- Occurs in moderate amount after breast stimulation

- No lump or other abnormality is found in either breast

Abnormal Physiological Discharge

There are conditions where the discharge has all the above characteristics but occurs throughout the month. The pituitary, thyroid, adrenal, and ovarian glands all release hormones that govern the production of breast fluid. If the thyroid gland is not producing enough hormones (hypothyroidism) it can lead to untimely production of breast milk. If you are having symptoms related to low thyroid function (fatigue, weight gain, dry skin, hair loss, cold intolerance, depression, irritability, abnormal menstrual cycles, decreased libido) along with breast discharge, inform your physician. Blood tests can determine if this is the cause, and medication can relieve symptoms.

Another condition causing excessive amounts of fluid from both breasts is called galactorrhea and is caused by elevated prolactin (the hormone that stimulates milk production) levels. Sometimes this condition occurs in combination with amenorrhea, the absence of menstrual periods. Often galactorrhea may be the result of a tumor in the pituitary gland. To check for this cause, prolactin levels can be measured in your blood; if the prolactin level is high, an MRI scan of the head can confirm or exclude the presence of a tumor. Medication may be prescribed to correct the problem or to block prolactin production. If you have a discharge that occurs in large amounts and you are not pregnant, contact your healthcare provider for evaluation of the underlying cause.

Discharge During Pregnancy

It is normal for pregnant women to have a bilateral discharge of breast fluid during pregnancy. However, some pregnant women may have a normal, spontaneous, usually bilateral, bloody-tinged discharge the last few months of pregnancy. This discharge is caused by high levels of progesterone and is usually not associated with disease. However, the physician should be notified and the breasts checked with a clinical exam. The discharge usually subsides shortly after delivery. If the discharge persists two months after delivery, further diagnostic testing should be performed.

Pharmacological Discharge

The use of some common medications **may** be the promoting cause of breast discharge that is the color of normal discharge—opaque to milky. Some drugs stimulate the breasts to produce breast fluid. If you have experienced a discharge and are presently using medications from one of the categories listed below, refer to Chapter 16, which includes a list of medications that may cause or promote breast discharge.

Many of the medications increase levels of prolactin, the hormone that stimulates milk production. This condition is **not harmful**, but your healthcare provider should be informed. If the amount is annoying, the medication may need to be changed or dosages adjusted.

Drug categories identified as possibly causing breast discharge:

Birth control pills
Hormones such as estrogen
Blood pressure medications
Narcotics or pain relievers
Psychiatric medications
Antidepressants
Gastrointestinal medications
Heart medications

Herbal Supplements

There has been an increase in reports of nipple discharge and breast pain with herbal dietary supplement use. These products may be marketed for weight loss, energy-increasing and ergogenic (performance enhancing) effects, PMS symptoms, menopausal symptoms, and bodybuilding. The herbs may also be present in teas and liquid diet formulas. Some liquid protein drinks use soybeans as their source of protein. Soy protein can have a hormonal effect on the breasts. If you notice a discharge after the use of supplements or liquid diet products, they may be the promoting factor. Two products that may cause breast discharge are Ginseng and Dong Quai.

Characteristics of Discharge Caused by Disease

We will discuss specific diseases that may cause a discharge in chapter 6. If your discharge has the following characteristics, consult your healthcare provider for a complete evaluation.

The discharge that concerns healthcare providers is usually:

■ **Persistent** throughout the month—does not vary with monthly cycle

■ **Spontaneous**—happens without squeezing the nipple or breast (you find it in your bra)

■ **Unilateral**—from one breast only, and usually from **one** or **several** duct openings on the nipple

■ **Abnormally colored**—clear and watery, clear and sticky (like an egg white), greenish-gray, or bloody in appearance (pink-tinged to red)

Factors increasing likelihood of disease in the breast producing discharge:

■ Lump in breast

■ Nipple inversion

■ Dimpling of skin

■ Redness or change of color of skin

■ Pain

Discharge Evaluation

The breast has approximately 6 to 10 openings on the nipple. Discharge can come from one or all of the duct openings. If you have a discharge, it is important to determine if the discharge is coming from one or multiple duct openings. Gently massage your breast and look closely at your nipple to determine how many duct openings produce discharge. Is the discharge coming from ducts located in more than one quadrant (1/4) of the nipple area or is it coming from one or two located close together in the same quadrant of the breast? This is an important first step in evaluating the cause.

Discharge from all the ducts, as well as both breasts, is usually due to physiological or pharmacological causes and is not clinically significant unless it occurs in large amounts throughout the month. Discharge from one or several ducts is most often from a change inside of a duct caused by disease, usually benign, but occasionally malignant. Worksheets designed to help you collect information on your discharge are located at the back of the book. This information will be helpful to your physician in evaluating the possible cause of your discharge.

The most specific diagnostic test used to evaluate breast discharge coming from one or several ducts is ductography (galactography). This procedure is performed in a breast center by a radiologist. The procedure starts with identifying the duct(s) producing the discharge. A small plastic cannula is inserted into the duct, allowing the physician to inject a dye into it. The breast is then imaged, and the radiologist looks at the film for anything inside of the duct that could cause any abnormal filling in the area. The physician may also use a clinical exam, cytology (study of cellular content of discharge), diagnostic mammography, or ultrasound to evaluate the discharge. If an abnormality is observed, the duct can be injected with a colored dye to mark it for surgical removal of the diseased duct only. Remember, the individual ducts and their lobe and lobular units do not interconnect with each other. They act as independent systems opening onto the nipple.

Remember:

- Understanding the kinds and causes of discharge will help you explain your discharge to your physician.

- Nipple discharge is not usually associated with cancer; but because it can be, **all nipple discharge needs to be evaluated**.

- Refer to tear-out worksheets on nipple discharge evaluation and for nipple discharge evaluation calendars.

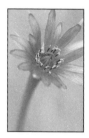

CHAPTER 6

COMMON BENIGN BREAST PROBLEMS

Breast Cysts

Cysts are fluid-filled sacs in the lobules that are relatively soft, round to oval in shape, and movable in the breast. A woman may have a single cyst or multiple cysts in one or both breasts. The size of a cyst can vary from very small microcysts to macrocysts which sometimes reach the size of a large egg. They are usually painless but may be painful if large, rapidly increasing in size, or pressing on a nerve. When you feel them, they may feel like water in a balloon under the skin. They occur at the end of the lobules in the milk-producing acini. Before a menstrual period, cysts usually increase in size and may become more painful. They can fill quickly with fluid, causing a lump that was not present at your last exam. Ultrasound may be used to distinguish the cyst from a solid mass. Most cysts occur in women between the ages of 30 and 50. Cysts are not common several years after menopause unless estrogen replacement therapy is taken. Ultrasound can usually confirm the diagnosis of a cyst because of the round, smooth appearance and their fluid make-up.

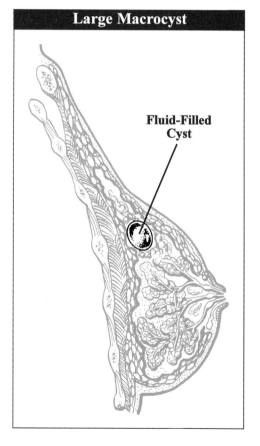

Large Macrocyst

Fluid-Filled Cyst

Galactocele

A galactocele is a cyst filled with breast milk. It occurs only in lactating women. The breast milk is blocked off in a duct. The area may feel lumpy in part of the breast, or it may feel like a distinct round or oval lump. The lump is usually firm, not tender, and is movable. Ultrasound can often confirm if the area is milk-filled. Aspiration may or may not be performed. If aspirated, the fluid obtained will be the color of breast milk. However, if the galactocele has been in the breast for a long period of time, the fluid may be thicker and darker. Galactoceles may require repeated needle aspirations, but surgery is rarely needed. Like other breast cysts, galactoceles are harmless.

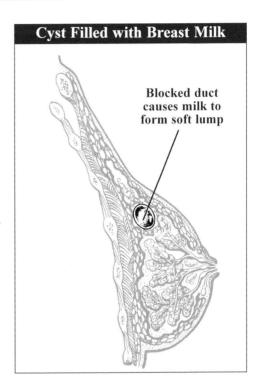

Cyst Filled with Breast Milk

Blocked duct causes milk to form soft lump

Cyst Aspiration

A physician will usually use a fine needle to aspirate (withdraw) the fluid from a cyst if it is large, palpable, painful, increasing in size, or if ultrasound is inconclusive. The needle is inserted, and the fluid is withdrawn into a syringe. This procedure may or may not be performed under ultrasound guidance. If the cyst disappears following aspiration and the fluid ranges from clear to dark yellow, or has a green, brownish, or sometimes even a bluish tint, the fluid is usually discarded. These are normal colors of breast fluid. The longer the fluid has been in the cyst, the darker the color. If the lump created by the cyst disappears completely and does not recur in six to eight weeks, no further evaluation is needed. If the fluid obtained has signs of blood (may be red from fresh blood or a brownish chocolate color from old blood) further evaluation of the cyst is needed. Follow-up may include a re-examination in several weeks, a mammogram, an ultrasound, or biopsy of the area.

Cysts are no longer considered a risk factor for breast cancer. Ducts become filled with old cells and become clogged, backing up fluid in the breast at the end of the ductal system where the fluid is produced. Cysts result from a normal aging process of the ducts in the breast, the result of filling and emptying over many years. A mere one percent of cysts have an occurrence of an intracystic papillary carcinoma. The good news is that this carcinoma does not spread past the lining of the cyst. Moreover, these occurrences are rare and are usually detected when a lump remains after aspiration or a bloody aspirate is obtained. Ultrasound can often identify their presence before aspiration.

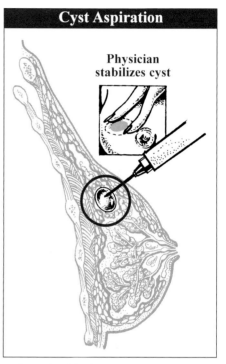

Cyst Aspiration

Physician stabilizes cyst

Reasons for aspiration are: (1) to confirm a lump is fluid-filled, (2) to prevent the cyst from hiding another change that could occur in the breast, (3) to reduce pain if the cyst is painful, and (4) to remove the presence of a palpable lump. Your healthcare provider will help you understand which cysts need to have aspiration performed.

Fibroadenoma

Fibroadenomas are solid, benign (noncancerous) tumors composed of fibrous and glandular tissues that are movable and not anchored in the surrounding breast tissues. They are the second most commonly occurring type of benign breast lump. Fibroadenomas occur most commonly between the ages of 20 and 40, but they can occur in even younger women. The lump is most often painless. It feels rubbery and firm because the outer rim has a dense collagen layer. Size may vary from a very small pea to a large lemon. There may be more than one lump in a single breast, or lumps may occur in both breasts. The hardness of the lump does not change during the menstrual cycle.

A fibroadenoma may be seen on a mammogram or ultrasound with characteristics that help identify it (smooth borders, round or lobulated). If mammography and ultrasound identify the characteristics of a fibroadenoma, a followup after six months may be recommended by some physicians. Other physicians prefer to perform a core biopsy for absolute confirmation and then observe the area for changes. Some studies have shown that approximately 50 percent of fibroadenomas disappear in several years. Others prefer to remove them surgically to prevent concealing any other change that could occur in the breast, or because the patient would rather have them removed.

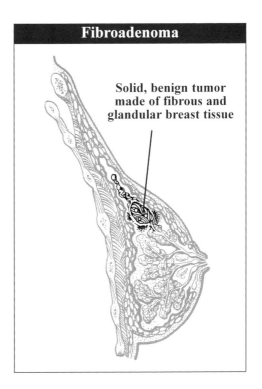

Fibroadenoma

Solid, benign tumor made of fibrous and glandular breast tissue

Phyllodes Tumors

Phyllodes (also spelled phylloides) tumors are usually benign tumors occurring in the glandular and connective tissue (stroma) of the breast. In rare cases they can be malignant. These rare types of tumor appear similar to a fibroadenoma but are differentiated by having an overgrowth of fibro-connective tissues. Because of their potential to become cancerous, the tumor is surgically removed with large margins.

Mammary Duct Ectasia

(Plasma Cell Mastitis or Periductal Mastitis)

Mammary duct ectasia is a condition that occurs most frequently in women immediately before and after menopause. It may occur in one, several or all of the ducts on one or both breasts. Ducts located beneath the nipple become filled and dilated with the cells that line the ducts. This occurs because of stagnation, and not because of a blockage. This accumulated debris appears as a thick, white to greenish-gray to blackish discharge from one, several or all of the nipple openings. The discharge can cause the nipple to itch and become irritated. The internal accumulation of debris in the duct can also cause a break in the cell walls (called mucosal ulceration) that can cause a bloody discharge. This ulceration causes the tissues around the ducts to swell from a chemical inflammatory reaction to the leaking fluid from inside the ducts. During this inflammatory progression of the condition, pain varies from mild to severe. The inflammation causes the tissues around the ducts to become fibrosed (thickened and hardened)

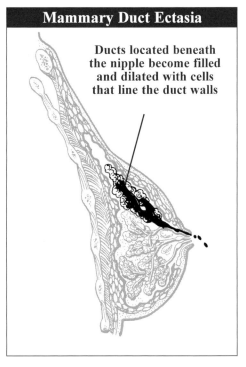

Mammary Duct Ectasia

Ducts located beneath the nipple become filled and dilated with cells that line the duct walls

and the nipple may retract as a result. The inflammation can develop into an infection (mastitis) and may even develop into an abscess (a localized collection of pus). Antibiotics will usually resolve the infection, but, occasionally, surgery is required to remove the abscessed duct(s). Mammary duct ectasia is not a cancerous condition. Smoking greatly increases the percentage of duct ectasia conditions that develop into chronic infections and abscesses. Duct ectasia can become a chronic problem with periods of remission and then exacerbations.

Fat Necrosis

Fat necrosis is the result of an injury to breast tissues that later becomes a benign (non-cancerous) lump. Fat necrosis happens occasionally after a hematoma (collection of blood from a bruise) forms following an injury or surgery. It may also occur in the area of a previous infection. The tissues die after the trauma, and gradually the breast forms a lump that is often difficult to distinguish from cancer because of its hardness and the fact that it may show microcalcifications on a mammogram. It may also cause skin retraction or dimpling. Often a biopsy is required to distinguish this benign lump from a cancerous tumor.

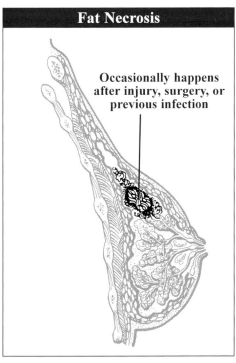

Fat Necrosis

Occasionally happens after injury, surgery, or previous infection

A very common cause of fat necrosis is injury caused by seatbelts during a car accident. The injury occurs when the seatbelt compresses the breast between the seatbelt and the ribs as the body is thrust forward with force. The typical injury is a furrowed deformed line across the breast. When the accident occurs it is most often accompanied with a hematoma (collection of blood) and edema (swelling). As this resolves, the injury can be seen on mammography as architectural changes, which are often accompanied with calcifications appearing in a band-like pattern in the breast. When fat necrosis of the tissues occur, retraction in the area may also be observed. These changes do not cause cancer, but would need to be evaluated by a healthcare provider.

Always inform your radiologist if you have been involved in an accident wearing a seatbelt and have experienced trauma to the breast.

Papilloma

Papillomas are benign, usually tiny, wart-like growths found in large ducts of the breast near the nipple area. They may occur as a single growth or in groups. Often a bloody discharge is seen coming from one duct opening on one nipple. The growths appear most often between the ages of 35 and 50. They are usually painless, unless multiple papillomas create a mass. Diagnosis is usually made by a ductogram (galactography), a procedure in which a cannula is inserted and radiographic dye is injected into the duct producing the discharge. X-ray pictures allow observation of the interior of the duct and can confirm the presence of an intraductal-filling defect. Papillomas are identified by the characteristic of being attached to the lining of the duct by a stalk (much like a mushroom). Surgery is required to remove the involved duct, even though it may not be cancerous, because of the bloody discharge and need for a definite diagnosis.

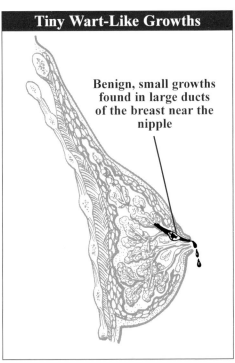

Tiny Wart-Like Growths

Benign, small growths found in large ducts of the breast near the nipple

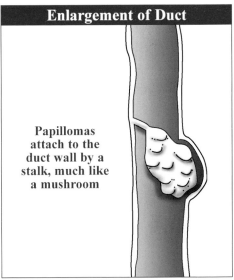

Enlargement of Duct

Papillomas attach to the duct wall by a stalk, much like a mushroom

Mastitis

Lactational mastitis is an inflammation that is most often seen in women who are breastfeeding. However, mastitis may occur at any time. Bacteria enter the breast, usually through the nipple, and invade the ducts. The bacteria cause localized areas of inflammation and infection, producing redness starting in one quadrant and accompanied by pain. The breast becomes swollen, tender and warm. Infection can quickly spread to other quadrants of the breast. A fever of 101° F and flu-like symptoms are common. The healthcare provider may perform a culture on the fluid from the breast to determine the exact cause.

Antibiotics are usually very effective in treating the infection and should be started as soon as symptoms appear. Symptoms usually improve two to three days after medication is started. However, the entire course of antibiotics prescribed by the healthcare provider should be taken. If the redness and pain does not respond to the antibiotics in several days, call your healthcare provider.

The infection may result in an abscess if not treated promptly with antibiotics. Occasionally, an abscess may require surgical drainage or removal. A healthcare provider will determine if a woman can continue to nurse during treatment for mastitis. Most providers agree that continuing to nurse can help clear the infection and is not harmful to the infant. However, for some women lactational mastitis may make it too painful to continue.

Pain can be managed with analgesics such as Tylenol®. It is important to wear a well-fitting bra during the day and night to prevent movement of the breast during the infection.

Women who have had mastitis or a breast abscess may have a texture change in the tissues or have a mammogram that shows microcalcifications (small particles seen on film) in the area of the previous infection. If you have had mastitis, write down which breast and what area of the breast was affected for your health records. Remind your healthcare provider of your history when you have your next mammogram. Being aware of your history will help the radiologist and could prevent unnecessary anxiety on your part if changes are observed on your film in this area of your breast.

Breast Abscess

About 10 percent of mastitis cases will form an abscess (a collection of pus) contained in one area of the breast. This area will feel hard, painful and warm to the touch. An abscess has a localized area of pain in one spot. Mastitis pain may be more generalized in the breast. Some abscesses will respond to antibiotic treatment if treatment is started early. However, some do not respond or may be too large or very painful. These will require that a healthcare provider drain the area surgically. Draining the abscess reduces pain immediately. Occasionally the healthcare provider may surgically remove the abscess. Because some abscesses tend to recur, some healthcare providers prefer surgical removal.

The most common site for breast abscesses is under the areola in the area of the ducts. Report any pain with tenderness and warmth of the tissues to a healthcare provider immediately so that treatment with antibiotics can be started.

Cellulitis

Cellulitis is an infection of the skin or connective tissues of the breast. It can occur when lymphatic drainage has been reduced by lymph node removal from surgery or radiation therapy. Women who have had lumpectomies have a potential to have cellulitis in the breast anytime after surgery. The same is true for women who have had a mastectomy; the chest wall is subject to infection. This condition is also common in diabetics and immunosuppressed individuals.

Infection starts in one area of the breast or chest wall, causing it to become tender, swollen, red, painful and warm to the touched. If left untreated, the infection can spread quickly. Fever and flu-like symptoms may occur.

Cellulitis needs immediate treatment with an antibiotic. After medication is started, symptoms usually improve in two to three days. However, all medication should be taken as prescribed. A well-fitted bra will help stabilize the breast and prevent pain caused by movement. Cellulitis can be recurrent and require treatment multiple times. Some physicians give women with a previous history of an infection a standing prescription to carry with them so an antibiotic can be started at the first sign of recurrence. Some infections require intravenous (IV) antibiotics because of their severity.

Mondor's Syndrome

Mondor's syndrome is an inflamed vein in the breast resulting from a clot. This rare condition may also be called "breast phlebitis" or "superficial periphlebitis." The condition may occur after trauma, muscular strain, radiation therapy, or surgical procedures. Often the cause is not found.

The inflamed vein will be painful and tender along its length. The area may feel like a thick cord in the breast. The pain may last from one to six weeks. However, you may be able to feel the cord-like vein for several months. The thickened vein may be visible on the surface of the breast. It may also cause skin retraction along the path of the vein. Because of these symptoms, a mammogram may be performed to confirm the absence of a coexisting malignancy.

Anti-inflammatory pain medication may be prescribed; no other treatment is necessary. When experiencing pain, a well-fitting bra should be worn day and night. The condition resolves itself over a period of time. Mondor's syndrome is a benign disease.

Sclerosing Adenosis

Sclerosing (hardening) adenosis (disease of a gland) is a condition that develops in the end of the lobules involving the acini, the part of the duct that produces milk or fluid. The fibrous tissues in this area begin to get larger and distort the lobular unit. Occasionally, this enlargement will combine with other enlarged acini and become large enough to produce an area that can be felt. The enlargement remains within the ducts and does not move outside of the lobular walls. This enlargement is called an adenosis tumor, a benign development in the breast.

Sclerosing adenosis is microscopic and is usually diagnosed when microcalcifications found on a mammogram are removed by a biopsy.

Shingles

(Herpes Zoster)

Shingles of the breast is rare but can occur. The condition is just like shingles on any other part of the body caused by the herpes zoster virus (chicken pox), and may also be recurrent. The outbreak is preceded by pain in the breast, fatigue, and fever. Small blisters occur on the skin in groups of 8 to 10 and are 2 - 3 mm (very small) in size. A healthcare provider will prescribe medication for pain and treatment of the virus, along with topical medications.

Other Conditions of the Breast:

Fungal Infections

The most common cause of redness and irritation under the folds of the breast is from the fungus *candida albicans*. Women with large pendulous breasts or women who work or exercise in warm climates are more likely to have a fungal irritation. The best treatment is to keep the area clean and dry. Oral or topical antifungal medications can be prescribed by a healthcare provider to treat the condition. Fungal conditions can be recurrent.

Infected Oil Gland

The oil glands (Montgomery's glands) surrounding the nipple may become clogged and an infection can occur. The breast, like other areas of skin on our body, may have pimples just like on the face. Treatment is usually an antibiotic cream applied topically. Occasionally a chronic infected gland may have to be surgically removed.

Remember:
■ Benign breast disease can cause many symptoms similar to cancer. Though these diseases are not life-threatening, it is important that you consult a healthcare provider and report any change or symptoms you experience.
■ Inform your radiologist or mammography technologist of any history of benign breast problems, needle aspirations, or surgical procedures when you have your mammogram. These areas could show up on your mammogram as microcalcifications or areas of change.

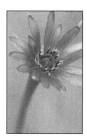

CHAPTER 7

WHAT YOUR HEALTHCARE PROVIDER NEEDS TO KNOW

Your healthcare provider is your partner in determining what is abnormal, what is not, and if you need further tests to help diagnose the finding. When you go to your healthcare provider for an exam of a breast change, you should be prepared to explain the following:

- date you found the lump or change

- time in your monthly cycle when the lump or change was found

- if the lump or change has been observed through a monthly cycle and if the characteristics have changed

- where you are in your monthly cycle on the day of your clinical exam

- location in the breast (if the lump is not easily found, find the lump and place the healthcare provider's hand in the area or explain the position you can best feel the lump; mark the area with an indelible ink pen before your visit)

- size of the lump when you found it (for example, the size of a pea or of a quarter)

- feel of the lump—whether it is hard, soft, painful, or non-painful

- any history of breast or ovarian cancer in your family, a personal history of any previous breast problems, or any other cancer

Your healthcare provider is your partner in guarding your breast health. Monitoring your breasts and reporting changes allows the healthcare provider to collect the evidence needed to make the best decisions about your breast care.

Communicating With Your Healthcare Provider

It is very important for you to feel comfortable talking with your healthcare provider about your breast health. Your questions and reports about what you have observed will help your provider give good advice and take the necessary steps to diagnose your problem. Some women find it difficult to feel comfortable discussing their breast health. However, it is important for you to find ways to feel comfortable in the relationship. Some suggestions for developing this relationship are as follows:

- Find a healthcare provider who is easy to talk with. Different people are attracted to different types of personalities. If you do not have a healthcare provider or you find it difficult to talk to your provider, ask a friend or a nurse to recommend someone.

- Be prepared for your office visit. Write down questions. Do not be embarrassed to bring a sheet of questions and ask that they be answered. This saves time and helps assure that your questions will be answered.

- Ask for written information and recommendations for educational literature, tapes, and videos. Learning the language and understanding more about your anatomy will make the communication process much easier between you and your healthcare provider.

- Ask if there is a nurse who would be able to answer any other questions should they come up after you leave. Often a healthcare provider will have a nurse already designated to provide this assistance.

- Be sure that you have the information necessary to provide a complete history for your chart. This record may be valuable to the healthcare provider when evaluating steps to take in a diagnostic decision process. (Personal history, family cancer history, medications, previous mammograms if seeing a new provider, previous biopsy reports, and a list of over-the-counter medications, vitamins or herbs.)

- Tell your healthcare provider how much you value his or her partnership with you in your health care. Remember, your healthcare providers also need positive feedback and appreciation. This can be valuable in keeping the lines of communication open.

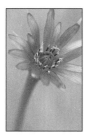

CHAPTER 8

DIAGNOSING YOUR PROBLEM

When you have a problem in your breast, your healthcare provider will first collect or review your medical history. A clinical breast exam will allow the doctor to feel or to see what you have found in your breast. To evaluate the findings, the healthcare provider may order a mammogram and/or an ultrasound, ductogram, or MRI. If an area is found that is suspicious, a biopsy may be required. Types of biopsies available are fine needle aspiration, core needle biopsy, stereotactic core needle biopsy, needle (wire) localization for a biopsy, methylene blue dye localization, incisional biopsy, and excisional biopsy. A brief explanation of each procedure follows.

Mammogram

A mammogram is an x-ray of the breast's internal structures. The breast is compressed with a paddle on a machine and pictures are made of each breast. Digital mammography is a newer type of procedure available in some facilities; however, it uses the same process except the pictures are sent to a computer instead of a film cassette. Quality is comparable.

There are two types of mammograms a healthcare provider may order. A **screening mammogram** is ordered when there are no known problems. Two pictures of each breast are taken. A **diagnostic mammogram** is ordered when there is a known problem such as a lump, pain, nipple discharge, or a change in color or rash of the skin. During a diagnostic mammogram, additional views may be taken including magnification views or spot compression of the area of concern.

A mammogram can detect lumps or signs of cancer years before they can be felt. Even though a mammogram has the ability to detect these changes, it cannot give an accurate diagnosis of what causes a change or whether the change is cancer. Some benign changes may appear similar to those of cancer. Mammography can also miss 10 - 15 percent of lumps in the breast. Therefore, mammography should always be combined with a clinical exam from a healthcare provider and supplemented by your breast self-exam.

If possible, go for a mammogram at the end of your menstrual period when the breasts are least tender so that the compression will be less uncomfortable. Wear separates so you can undress from the top only. Do not wear perfume, deodorant, powder, or oil on the day of the procedure. These substances could cause artifacts (debris) to show up on the film, requiring further evaluation.

A common complaint about the mammogram procedure is discomfort from compression. A paddle to flatten your breast tissue applies compression. Compression is necessary to spread the breast tissues as thin as possible, to keep the breast tissues from moving during the exam and to minimize the amount of radiation received. Compression helps provide the clearest image possible so that the radiologist can see all the details of your tissues clearly, improving the accuracy of the mammogram. Compression only lasts for a few seconds, during which time there may be some discomfort, but normally not pain. If you experience pain, tell your technologist.

A radiologist will interpret the films, and a report will be sent to you and your healthcare provider. Ask when you can expect to receive this report and who will talk to you about it if you have a mammogram that shows an abnormality.

A Questionable Mammography Report . . . What Does This Mean?

If you have a screening mammogram and something is found, a repeat exam may be needed. However, there are other reasons for a repeat mammogram request such as suboptimal positioning, inadequate exposure of the film, or artifacts (unwanted objects found on the picture—for example, spots caused by deodorant). For many different reasons, the radiologist may issue a report requesting additional film or studies and ask you to come back for a diagnostic mammogram for further evaluation. The three main changes the radiologist is looking for are calcifications, masses, and architectural distortion (changes in the normal tissue structures).

- A mass is any group of cells clustered together more densely than the surrounding tissue. The size, shape, and margins (edges) of the mass help the radiologist evaluate the likelihood of cancer.

- Calcifications are tiny mineral deposits within the breast tissue that appear as small white specks on the mammogram films.

- Architectural distortion is a change in the normal structural pattern of breast tissue that a radiologist often detects by comparing one breast film to the other.

If you receive or have received a report requesting your return because of what has been found on your mammogram, remember that there are causes other than breast cancer. In fact, the majority of areas re-evaluated by radiologists are not cancerous. Be assured that your radiologist is exercising caution to protect your health by requesting additional pictures or procedures. It may help if you talk to the radiologist or to a mammographic technologist and ask for an explanation of what they have found and how they plan to further evaluate your breast(s).

The Diagnostic Mammogram

Diagnostic mammography is different from screening mammography in that additional views of the breast are taken (screening mammography has two views of each breast). Diagnostic mammography is more time-consuming and usually costs more than screening mammography, because it is a tailored exam based on your findings. The goal of diagnostic mammography is to define the exact size and location of the breast abnormality and to provide an image of the surrounding tissues and lymph nodes.

Additional types of pictures (spot compression or magnification views) may be taken of an area that has an unknown abnormality. Spot compression is usually performed to further assess a lump or mass. A smaller compression paddle is placed directly over the area found, allowing the radiologist to examine more closely the characteristics of the areas. Magnification views enlarge an area for closer viewing by the radiologist. This is particularly helpful when microcalcifications have been found. Magnification allows the radiologist to carefully examine the characteristics of the calcifications to determine if they have benign or malignant characteristics. In many cases, close-up views or spot compression alone will show that the abnormality is most likely non-cancerous (benign).

To help the radiologists readily identify an area warranting closer examination, skin markers (similar to a Band-Aid or a small BB-like metal ball) may be placed on the breast if an abnormality is seen on a previous film or a lump can be felt. The markers do not hide any breast tissue. They may also be placed over moles or scars to mark the area for the radiologist.

What Are Calcifications?

One of the most common reasons for patient recall is **calcifications**. Calcifications may be micro (small) or macro (large). Calcifications are caused by calcium deposits left by cells when they die. You may think of them as the "ashes" of dead cells. They are caused by natural aging of the breast, an injury to your breast, cysts or cyst aspirations, mastitis, abscesses, duct ectasia, scar tissue, or other benign (non-cancerous) causes; they can also be a sign of cancer. They are not related to calcium from your diet. Microcalcifications are the smallest particles that can be seen on mammography film (less than 1/50 of an inch). They appear as small white specks, looking much like dust on the film.

Because calcifications may be signs of cancer, the radiologist will carefully study any found on your film. About half of all cancers diagnosed by mammography are found as a cluster of microcalcifications. The radiologist will look closely with a magnifying glass at the shape, the size and the number found in a certain area, and the spacing to see if they are grouped together or if they follow the outline of a duct (signs of ductal carcinoma in situ). The individual shape of each calcification will also be evaluated closely. Different shapes are associated with different causes. If there is clustering, or if the individual shapes or sizes of the calcifications are suspicious, the radiologist will order additional studies and may request a followup exam in several months. Approximately 90 percent of ductal carcinoma in situ, the earliest form of cancer, is found by mammography alone in this manner.

Breast Density

The glandular tissues of the breast (ducts, lobes, lobules) are where breast disease begins. Because they are under the skin, mammography is needed to image the internal structure to detect any abnormalities. The glands and fibrous connective tissues are dense and show up white, whereas the fatty tissues are dark on a mammogram. Young women tend to have denser breasts and older women more fatty ones. However, density varies with your own unique breast composition. Breast masses also appear white, like glandular and connective tissues, on mammography and may be camouflaged. The denser the normal tissues are, the more likely this is to occur. After menopause, the glands in the breasts tend to become replaced by fat, making abnormal masses easier to detect with mammography. This is one reason regular mammography is started at forty (unless a woman is at high risk of developing breast cancer) and is also the reason that ultrasound may be used when a change is detected in younger women.

The American College of Radiology has developed a four-level grading system to categorize breast density on a scale of 1 (fatty) to 4 (most dense). They conducted a study on breast density and reported, "We find dense breast approximately 66 percent of the time in premenopausal women, 25 percent of the time in postmenopausal women not taking hormones, and in 50 percent of postmenopausal women taking hormones."

For this reason, annual mammography after the age of forty and a clinical exam are recommended to detect any changes early.

The Return Visit

If you have received a report that asks for further evaluation of your breasts and feel anxious about the visit, you may want to call and request an earlier return appointment. It may also help to ask to speak to the radiologist or technologist about the reasons for your recall visit. Ask what additional tests or procedures to expect on your return visit and for written materials to help you understand your condition. You may also ask a friend or a mate to accompany you on the visit. Having someone with you will help reduce the stress. Managing your fears during this time is very important. On the day of your return appointment, inform the radiologist if you have a history of injury, infection, or benign disease in this breast. It is also very important, if your previous mammograms were not performed in the same facility, that you get your previous film for comparison by the radiologist. Comparison with a previous film is an important factor for the radiologist to give the best interpretation of the new finding.

Additional Diagnostic Tests

Mammography is the best screening tool we have for breast cancer, but it cannot tell for certain if the identified abnormality is cancerous or benign. Additional tests may be ordered to help the radiologist make a diagnosis. Imaging tests that may be used in addition to mammography are ultrasound and breast MRI (Magnetic Resonance Imaging).

Ultrasound

An ultrasound is a procedure that uses sound waves instead of x-rays to visualize the internal structures of the breasts. The Food and Drug Administration (FDA) does not approve the use of ultrasound as a screening tool by itself because it cannot detect microcalcifications, is highly operator dependent, and has no way of telling if the whole breast has been scanned. Therefore, an ultrasound is usually ordered to further characterize findings observed on a mammogram or breast exam. The healthcare provider can usually tell from this test whether the area is filled with fluid (a cyst) or is a solid lump. It may also be used first if you are pregnant or younger than 25. Ultrasound is also used for guidance in cyst aspirations, needle or core biopsies, pre-operative needle localizations, or other procedures.

There is no preparation for ultrasound, and it is painless. An instrument that resembles a microphone is slowly passed over your breast after a jelly-like substance is applied. Sound waves are reflected off the internal organs and an image mapped out by the echo is produced on a screen being viewed by the healthcare provider. The exam takes from 5 - 20 minutes.

Though most true breast lumps will be found by mammography and ultrasound, some abnormalities escape detection on both imaging tests. For example, a lump may be able to be felt but will not appear on mammography or ultrasound images. If a palpable change in the breast identified by a healthcare provider is questionable, even with a negative mammography and ultrasound, the radiologist may still recommend a needle biopsy of the area.

Breast MRI (Magnetic Resonance Imaging)

The FDA approved breast MRI in 1991 as a supplemental tool (additional test) to mammography to help diagnose breast cancer. Radiologists often use a dedicated MRI machine to further investigate breast concerns first detected with mammography; or during a physical exam to clarify or verify recommendations concerning abnormalities. It is also an excellent imaging tool for women with implants for augmentation (enlargement) because it can show the breast tissues surrounding the implant that might be obscured with mammography. MRI is also useful in determining what stage the breast cancer is in by imaging the nodes between the ribs and below the clavicle (collarbone). It is now being investigated as a screening tool in high-risk younger women identified by a strong family risk or by their carrying a mutated BRCA1 and BRCA2 (BR=breast, CA=cancer) gene.

Benefits of MRI:

- Evaluation of breast implants for ruptures or leaks and evaluation of breast tissues behind implants
- Effective in imaging dense breasts and young high-risk women's breasts
- Evaluation of inverted nipples for evidence of cancer
- Evaluation to determine if lumpectomy or mastectomy is the best surgical choice. May detect areas not seen by mammography and ultrasound.
- Evaluation for recurrence of breast lumps in lumpectomy breast
- Effective in locating primary tumors not seen on mammography if positive lymph nodes are present

Limitations of MRI:

- Costs ten times more than mammography
- Takes approximately four times longer
- Cannot identify microcalcifications
- Requires injection of contrast agent into a vein before exam
- Problems distinguishing between cancerous and non-cancerous tumors
- Advanced, dedicated MRI equipment is often not available in smaller centers and is usually limited to larger centers having the equipment needed to localize or mark a lesion located on MRI for biopsy or surgical removable.

Galactography or Ductography

To evaluate a nipple discharge, your radiologist may use galactography (ductography) if the discharge is from one or two openings on a breast. The nipple is cleansed with a cloth to remove plugs of keratin (wax-like substance) that close the nipple openings. Using a magnifying glass, a very fine plastic or metal catheter is threaded into the duct identified as having the discharge. A contrast agent is injected into the duct to allow it to be visualized on mammography so it can be observed for any abnormality that causes a defect in the filling of the duct. If a disease is found, the duct may also be marked with dye to visibly identify it for a surgeon. Identifying the duct and dye-marking it allows the diseased duct only to be removed during surgery, saving healthy breast tissues and improving cosmetic outcomes.

Breast Biopsy

Imaging procedures only tell us when there is an abnormal finding in the breast. Only when we have a tissue specimen evaluated by a pathologist using a microscope can we have a definite diagnosis. Areas that have cancer characteristics on imaging may be benign and those that have benign characteristics may be cancerous. Therefore, a biopsy for an accurate diagnosis is always needed. This tissue can be sampled using one of numerous biopsy procedures.

Biopsy Types

The most appropriate method should be selected according to the characteristics and location of the abnormality. We will explain the least invasive first and continue to the methods that are most invasive.

Biopsy Type	Selection Criteria	Size of Biopsy Specimen	Anesthetic Required	Advantages	Disadvantages
Fine Needle Aspiration (FNA)	Cyst or palpable solid lesion. Lesions seen on ultrasound	22-25 gauge needle. 2-6 sections of solid lesion sampled	None with simple cyst. Local with solid lesion	Quickest diagnosis. No stitches or scar	Small sample. Requires cytopathologist to read sample. Skill of provider can be a limitation
Core Needle (No image guidance)	Solid lesion	10-14 gauge coring needle	Local	Larger sample. No stitches or minimal scar	Multiple needle insertions. Potential to sample wrong area without imaging
Core Needle (Image guidance using Ultrasound or Stereotactic)	Solid lesions. Calcifications	10-14 gauge coring needle. 1/4" skin incision for instrument insertion (optional)	Local	Larger sample. No stitches or minimal scar. Imaging increases accuracy	Multiple insertions of needle
Vacuum Assisted Core Biopsy (Mammotome or MIBB)	Solid lesions. Calcifications	11-14 gauge needle. 1/4" skin incision for instrument insertion (optional)	Local	Can remove calcifications. One insertion of biopsy instrument to collect multiple solid core samples	Clinician skill dependent. Location of lesion in breast (not near chest wall or in very small breast)
Large Core (ABBI)	Solid lesions. Calcifications	5-20 mm of solid breast tissue (size of wine cork)	Local	Provides large sample similar to surgical biopsy	Removes healthy tissue between skin and lesion - Stitches and scar. Hematoma potential increase. Increased recovery time
Surgical Biopsy	Solid lesions. Calcifications (wire localized). Lesions close to chest wall	Requires 1-2" incisions or larger	Heavy Sedation. General Anesthesia	Largest tissue sample	Longer recovery. Stitches and scar. Complications from anesthesia. Future mammography interpretation

69

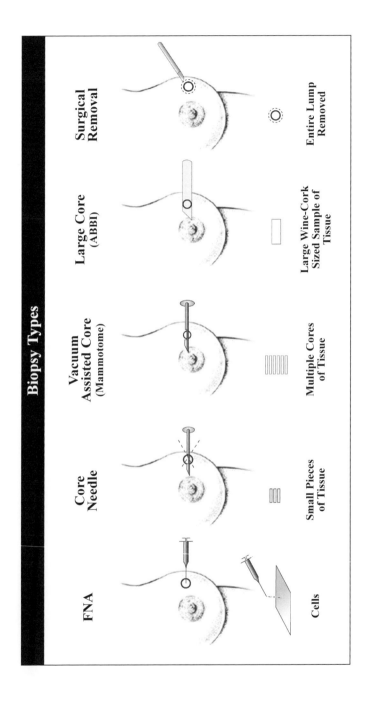

Biopsy Risks Increase As Method
Becomes More Invasive

TYPE OF BIOPSY	RISK SCALE 1 (least) - 5 (greatest)
Fine Needle Aspiration Biopsy	1
Core Needle Biopsy	2
Vacuum-Assisted Biopsy (Mammotome)	3
Large Core Biopsy (ABBI)	4
Open Surgical Biopsy	5

Risks of minimally invasive biopsies include:

■ Bruising

■ Potential for hematoma (collection of blood in site)

■ Potential for infection

■ Scarring is rare unless the procedure requires stitches to close the area

Requirements and risks of surgical biopsies include:

■ Requires procedure be performed in a surgical suite

■ Requires intravenous sedation and/or anesthesia

■ Requires stitches and leaves a scar on the breast

■ May change the appearance of the breast if a large amount of tissue is removed

■ May require wire localization to mark the area for the surgeon (performed under mammography or ultrasound to locate lesion) prior to surgery

■ Increased risk of bleeding and infection

■ Risk of hematoma (collection of blood) or seroma (collection of fluid in area)

■ Increased pain from more extensive procedure and longer recovery time

For core and surgical biopsies, you should inform your physician if you are taking aspirin, ibuprofen, blood thinners, or herbal supplements on a regular basis. After a biopsy, you should report any sudden or severe pain, the appearance of a lump in the area of the biopsy, or any redness or discharge at the incisional site. Any elevation of temperature over 101° F should also be reported immediately.

FNA (Fine Needle Aspiration) Biopsy

Fine needle aspiration is the insertion into the lump of a small-gauge needle with an attached empty syringe. FNA can be used to determine if a lump is filled with fluid or is solid. It can also be used to biopsy a solid lump by aspirating cells in different areas of the lump that are sent to a cytopathologist (a pathologist who identifies disease by cell samples). If fluid is withdrawn into the syringe, the lump is a cyst. Fluid from a cyst considered to be benign (not cancerous) is usually light to dark yellow or greenish and is normally discarded. Fluid that resembles chocolate milk or has obvious blood in it needs evaluation by cytology (identification of type of cells that make up the fluid). It is possible that the needle can puncture a small blood vessel causing bright red blood in fluid. Cysts are a normal occurrence in women approaching menopause and are no longer considered a pre-condition for cancer.

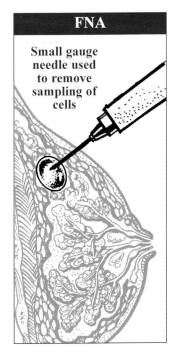

FNA

Small gauge needle used to remove sampling of cells

Core Needle Biopsies

Free Hand Core

Core needle biopsy is also called percutaneous (through the skin) biopsy and involves removing small samples of breast tissue using a hollow (core) needle. It is similar to FNA, but a larger coring needle is used. One method is a freehand procedure. This is for lumps that can be felt. The healthcare provider stabilizes the lump with one hand and inserts the coring biopsy instrument with the other.

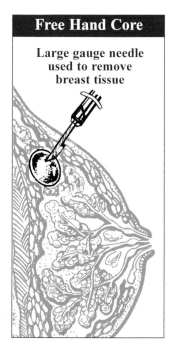

Free Hand Core

Large gauge needle used to remove breast tissue

The area biopsied is cleansed and injected with lidocaine to anesthetize it where the needle will be inserted. Pressure may be felt, but pain should be minimal. Three to six separate core needle insertions are typically needed to obtain a sufficient sample of breast tissue. The tissues removed are sent to a laboratory for evaluation by a pathologist.

Ultrasound Guided Core

Core biopsies can be performed using ultrasound as an imaging guidance tool to locate the abnormality. The physician locates the area with ultrasound and guides the biopsy needle to obtain the core samples. Ultrasound allows visualization of the area and the needle throughout the procedure. Still pictures can be made during the procedure.

Stereotactic Core Biopsy

Stereotactic biopsy is a core biopsy using specialized equipment that allows the radiologist to take a series of mammography films, locate the biopsy area on a computer, and then calculate where the needle should be inserted. This biopsy procedure is used for areas that cannot be felt but were identified in the breast by mammography, such as microcalcifications. A small surgical nick in the skin may be made to insert the instrument but usually no stitches are required. Stereotactic procedures may be performed with the woman either sitting up or lying on her abdomen (a special table allows a woman's breasts to fall through an opening in the table). The breast is compressed and visualized by mammography to allow the radiologist to relocate the suspicious area found previously on the mammography film. Medication is injected to numb the breast. Tissue samples are removed and sent to the laboratory where a pathologist studies the tissues and sends a report to your healthcare provider. The test requires from 30 minutes to one hour. When completed, a bandage is placed over the area, and the patient is allowed to return to her normal activities if they are not strenuous. No scar is left on the breast.

Vacuum Assisted Core Biopsy
(Brand names: Mammotome or MIBB)

Unlike other core methods that require repeated insertions of the needle, vacuum-assisted biopsy allows for the removal of multiple tissue samples with only one insertion of the biopsy instrument through a small surgical nick made in the skin. The biopsy probe is positioned in the area of the abnormality. The probe has a vacuum line that pulls the breast tissue into the sampling chamber. A rotating cutting device collects the tissue and carries it back to a tissue collection area in the probe. The physician can then rotate the probe without withdrawing it from the breast and collect another sample. The procedure is repeated until approximately 8 - 12 cores are obtained. When the core samples are completed, the probe is removed and pressure is applied to the site. A small sterile clip may be placed into the biopsy site to mark the location in case a future biopsy or mammogram of the area is needed. This microclip is left inside the breast and causes no pain, disfigurement, or harm. A sterile bandage is placed over the site. If needed, Tylenol® and ice packs applied to the area may be used to reduce pain after the procedure. The breast may appear bruised and be sore for a week after the biopsy.

Large Core Biopsy

(Advanced Breast Biopsy Instrumentation—ABBI)

ABBI is a large core surgical biopsy procedure that uses an instrument that removes an entire lesion in one piece. The procedure is performed under image guidance (stereotactic) on a biopsy table with the patient lying face down. A local anesthetic is injected while the breast is maintained in compression. The biopsy instrument is inserted and removes a piece of breast tissue (including skin, healthy breast tissues, and the lesion) approximately the size of a wine cork. Because of the large size of the sample taken, stitches are usually required to close area. The breast may appear bruised and be sore for a week or two after the biopsy.

Incisional Biopsy

An incisional biopsy is the removal of a small piece of the lump or suspicious area under local (numbing the breast only) or general (put to sleep) anesthesia. A surgeon cuts the sample from the breast. The sample is sent to the laboratory for evaluation by a pathologist, and a report is sent to the surgeon. Before surgery, depending on the healthcare provider, a pre-admission work-up will be required, consisting of blood work, medical history, an electrocardiogram, or other procedures. After surgery, the patient will be sent to outpatient recovery to be monitored and then allowed to return home. Restrictions on activities will vary according to the extent of the biopsy. Pain can usually be managed with Tylenol®. However, the breast will be sore for several days. Normal activities can usually be resumed in several days or when the stitches are removed.

Excisional Biopsy

Excisional biopsy is the removal of an entire lump or suspicious area by a surgeon (in a surgical room) under general or local anesthesia. Depending on the healthcare provider, a pre-admission work-up will be required before surgery, including blood work, a medical history, an electrocardiogram or other procedures. The area surrounding the lump, referred to as the **margins**, may be removed at the same time. The size of the incision varies according to the size of the lump removed, and the area is closed with several stitches. After surgery, the patient remains in outpatient recovery to be monitored and is then allowed to return home. Pain can usually be controlled with oral medications, such as Tylenol® or a prescription ordered by your physician, after returning home. Most healthcare providers allow patients to resume normal activities (depending on the extent of the surgery) in several days. Soreness usually lasts a week or two, and a return visit must be made for stitches to be removed. A pathologist will study the tissue, and a report will be sent to the referring healthcare provider.

Procedures Used in Conjunction With Surgical Biopsy

Needle (Wire) Localization

Needle localization is a procedure that is performed with mammography or ultrasound to mark a suspicious area that is not palpable for surgery, using a needle to insert a fine wire. The radiologist locates the suspicious area on the x-ray or ultrasound screen and then places one to several fine wires into the area of the lesion. Bracketing means that two or more wires are placed to mark the edges (margins) of an entire lesion so that the surgeon can remove the entire area that was visible during mammography, but not visible during surgery. The patient remains awake during the localization procedure. Usually, medication to numb the area of the breast is given. The wires are taped to the breast after placement and the patient is taken to surgery. The mammography films showing the final placement of the wires will be available for the surgeon. The surgeon sometimes requires the patient be put to sleep for the surgery. If the area was localized for microcalcifications, the removed tissue will be x-rayed to determine if microcalcifications are present before the surgery is completed. The specimen removed is sent to a laboratory to be evaluated by a pathologist, and a report is sent to your healthcare provider.

Methylene Blue Dye Localization

Methylene blue dye localization is a procedure during which a radiologist locates the suspicious area under mammography and injects a blue dye through a needle to mark the area. The blue dye identifies the area that the surgeon will remove during surgery. During the dye insertion, the patient is awake. The surgeon sometimes requires that the patient be put to sleep during the surgery. The area removed is sent to a laboratory to be evaluated by a pathologist, and a report is sent to your healthcare provider.

Questions To Ask Before Your Biopsy

Sometimes it is impossible for a healthcare provider to rule out disease without the use of a biopsy. Having a biopsy protects your health by helping your healthcare team determine for sure what is in your breast. One-step procedures—when surgery is performed at the time of the biopsy, if cancer is found—are rarely done today. Two-step procedures—biopsy first and surgery later—are now the preferred method. This additional step gives time to consider all options. You may wish to ask the following questions before your biopsy:

■ What type of biopsy will I have?

■ Will the procedure be done as an outpatient in your office, at a hospital, or at a surgical center?

■ Will this surgery require wire or methylene blue localization before surgery to mark the area?

■ Can I continue to take any regular medications prior to procedure?

■ Will I need any special tests before the procedure? (blood studies, electrocardiogram, etc.)

■ What type of anesthesia will you use—local or general? (You could be put to sleep for an excisional biopsy.)

■ Will I need to have someone drive me home?

■ Is there any preparation on my part? (no eating, drinking, etc.)

■ How long should the biopsy take?

■ Will I have any stitches? (for ABBI, incisional, or excisional biopsy)

■ Will there be any special care of the area after the biopsy? (dressings to change, special cleansing of the area, bathing instructions)

■ Should I expect to have pain in the area after the biopsy? If so, what should I take to control the pain?

■ Will I need a return appointment for an evaluation of the area?

■ When can I return to my normal activities after the biopsy?

■ When will I hear, and who will give me the results of the pathology report?

Biopsy Anxiety

Women often report after a breast biopsy that the most painful part of the procedure was waiting for the final diagnosis from the pathology report, not the biopsy procedure. Not knowing if the area in their breast is cancerous can create high levels of stress. Anxiety is normal for most women. However, there are things you can do to help reduce your anxiety if you require a biopsy.

- Ask your healthcare providers how long it will take to be scheduled to have your biopsy and how long it will take to receive your biopsy report. If this time frame is unacceptable to you psychologically, tell them how worried you are and how important it is for you to find out your results in a more timely manner. Many hospitals and breast centers specialize in providing a timely biopsy and biopsy results to reduce this anxiety, although they know the vast majority will be benign. They offer this service because they recognize that the psychological pain created by waiting is so great for women.

- It is also helpful to remember that most breast cancers have been growing for years and are just now identified. Taking several weeks to look into a second opinion and select your healthcare team is not going to endanger your health.

- Ask if your breast center has a nurse specializing in education and support. Call her and ask the questions that are important to you. Ask for written information on all procedures and on your final diagnosis.

- Take a friend or partner with you for the procedure. Sharing this time with someone reduces some of the anxiety and allows someone else to hear what your healthcare team tells you.

If you find your anxiety overwhelming, ask for medication to calm your nerves before the procedure. Psychological suffering needs attention from a healthcare provider the same as physical suffering. Talk to your healthcare team about your needs and fears.

Remember:

- The biopsy wait-period has the highest amount of patient anxiety for most women; seek out a center that will provide you education and support during this time, and provide you with a timely diagnosis.

CHAPTER 9

YOUR BIOPSY ANSWER: THE PATHOLOGY REPORT

If a biopsy is required to diagnose a suspicious lump or change, the removed tissues will be sent to the pathology (study of disease) laboratory where the tissues are evaluated by a pathologist (physician who identifies disease) to determine if they are malignant (cancerous) or benign (not cancerous). The pathology report will be sent to the referring physician, who should then contact you. The amount of time between your biopsy and getting the results depends on the type of studies ordered. You should ask your physician how long it should take to hear your results.

What You Need to Know About Your Biopsy Report

When you receive your report, you will want to clarify the following:

- What was the name of the cell type of the lump or abnormality removed?
- Was it malignant (cancerous) or benign (non-cancerous)?
- If benign, will this condition recur?
- Will I need any additional surgery?
- Are there any options besides surgery to treat this condition?
- Within what time frame do I need to have the surgery performed?
- What type of surgery is required?
- Do I have any surgical options?
- If further surgery is required, will there be any followup treatment?
- Do you recommend a change in diet or medication for the condition?
- What additional signs or symptoms should I watch for and report to a healthcare provider?

- How often will I need to have a clinical exam by a physician?
- What schedule is recommended for my future mammograms?
- Is this condition hereditary? Are my children at increased risk?

Some pathologists welcome the opportunity to explain more about your pathology report. If you would like to speak to your pathologist, ask your healthcare provider.

Remember:

- A lump or change in the breast may warrant a breast biopsy to determine if it is benign or malignant

- Your physician will determine the most appropriate type of biopsy for your abnormality

- Minimally invasive biopsies carry fewer potential complications and can be performed with only local anesthesia

- Surgical biopsies are sometimes required because of the location of the abnormality in the breast or other characteristics of the abnormality

- Approximately 80 percent of biopsies performed are benign (not cancerous)

- Discuss all options to diagnose your abnormality with your healthcare provider and ask for written information on the recommended procedure

- Ask what laboratory your biopsy specimen will be sent to, when the final report will be ready, and who will most likely give you the final diagnosis

- Ask for a written copy of your pathology report

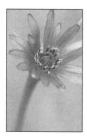

CHAPTER 10

RISKS FROM HORMONES AND DIET

The media constantly presents information on the causes of breast cancer. Most recently the subjects of diet and hormones have been topics hotly discussed. Often the message is frightening. It is difficult to sort out what really increases risk for breast cancer.

Many women look at the risk factors listed in the literature for breast cancer—early menstruation, late menopause, first pregnancy after age 30, no children, and family history of cancer—identify with one or more of the stated risk factors and live a life clouded with fear because they think that they are at high risk. These risk factors are facts over which women have little or no control. What is even more important to remember is that 76 percent of the women who had breast cancer in the past few years had none of the listed risk factors. Depending on the stated risk factors is not a good idea, because doing so can cause you to overestimate or underestimate your own personal risk. Having no risk factors may create a false sense of protection, while having risk factors may cause you to become fearful and suffer emotional distress from worrying about future breast cancer.

To compound these fears, the topics of diet, birth control and supplemental estrogen therapy are highly debated as being additional risk factors. This creates anxiety for many women when deciding to take hormonal medications.

The goal of this book is to help you reach a healthy balance in assessing your risk through looking at the latest information on controversial influences. All women are at risk for breast cancer. So we all have to take balanced steps to protect ourselves. Creating balance in our approach to breast health comes from understanding how our breasts function, how to monitor for changes, and how to enter into a partnership with a healthcare provider to help in this task.

No one really knows what causes breast cancer. Many factors have been suggested and clinical trials have proven that certain factors may cause women to be more susceptible. The problem is that these studies constantly offer conflicting data. One study will say that something may be a promoting factor, and another will say that it is not. The best approach is to depend on your healthcare provider for the latest information. The major questions women ask about protecting their breast health mostly concern the areas where they can make personal decisions to influence their health.

Hormonal Medications

Women are often concerned and confused about the relationship between breast cancer and the use of hormonal medications to prevent pregnancy and treat menopausal symptoms. The latest average of all studies reveals that there is only a slight (1 to 2 percent) increase in risk and this has to be compared to increased benefits in health and quality of life. Many of the studies causing these fears were done years ago when the medications prescribed had much higher levels of hormones. Birth control pills and estrogen supplements are now prescribed using the lowest dosages possible. The Hormone Foundation reports that oral contraceptives prescribed now contain one-fourth of the estrogen and one-tenth of the progestin dose of earlier pills. Using hormonal medication is an individual decision, and only after consultation with your healthcare provider can a choice be made that is right for you.

Oral Contraceptives

(Birth Control)

The use of birth control pills prevents unwanted pregnancies, but may also be prescribed to reduce breast pain and relieve symptoms of the peri-menopausal transition. In the past, studies about the use of oral contraceptives and their relationship to the incidence of breast cancer varied among study conclusions. Recently, a lot of questions about oral contraceptives and future breast cancer risks were answered when a study involving a total of 9,257 women was published in the *New England Journal of Medicine* on June 27, 2002. Out of these women, 4575 had breast cancer and 4682 did not have breast cancer. Both groups were interviewed about oral contraceptive use. The results were: 77 percent of the cancer patients and 79 percent of the cancer-free women had taken some type of oral contraceptive.

Dr. Robert Spirtas, Chief of Contraception/Reproductive Health, National Institute of Child Health and Human Development commented on the study: "It was a chance to look at women over a lifetime to see what the risk has been."

The *New England Journal of Medicine* summarized the author's conclusions of the study: "Those who had never taken the pill were about as likely to have breast cancer as those who were taking it or had taken it. It did not matter whether they were black or white; whether they were fat, skinny, or of average weight; whether they took the early variety of the pill containing high doses of hormones, or a later, lower-dose pill; or whether they had a family history of breast cancer, had gone through menopause or started taking contraceptives before they were 20. Among women from 35 to 64 years of age, current or former oral-contraceptive use was not associated with a significantly increased risk of breast cancer"

"I think that what was impressive was that, no matter which way you looked at the data, no matter which subset, the result was null. It's nice to be able to give good news to women about something so many women take or have taken," reported Dr. Kathy J. Helzlsouer, Cancer Specialist, Epidemiology, Johns Hopkins University School of Public Health.

This study helped reduce the fear felt by women taking oral contraceptives about their increased risk of breast cancer and is also helpful for those debating about using oral contraceptives in the future.

Hormone Replacement Therapy

Most women go through the menopausal transition of life experiencing some or all of the symptoms associated with reduced female hormones. Symptoms include:

- Hot flashes, night sweats

- Vaginal dryness, causing itching and painful intercourse

- Osteoporosis, increasing risk of broken bones

- Mood swings, nervousness, and irritability

- Frequent urination, painful urination, and stress incontinence (leaking urine when coughing, laughing, or when bladder is full)

- Insomnia

Estrogen replacement therapy reduces these side effects and recent studies have shown that it may also provide some protective effects/benefits with Alzheimer's disease, diabetes, and cataracts.

Hormone replacement may consist of a combination of estrogen and progesterone (HRT = hormone replacement therapy) or estrogen alone (ERT = estrogen replacement therapy). Women with an intact uterus are often prescribed estrogen with progesterone to reduce the incidence of uterine cancer. Women with no uterus are most often prescribed estrogen alone.

There are many non-hormonal therapies that can address menopausal symptoms. Discuss with your healthcare provider other treatments available, including herbal products that may be more appropriate for you. In this section we address the risks and fears associated with hormonal treatments.

Clinical Study of Hormone Use

The study creating the most interest lately about hormones and breast cancer was the Women's Health Initiative (WHI) Study released in July 2002. The study was conducted on women ages 50 - 79 with an intact uterus. Women were given either Prempro (a combination of Premarin and Provera) or a placebo (tablet with no medication). Prempro is a combination of two drugs; Premarin is .625 mg conjugated equine estrogen (derived from pregnant horses' urine), plus Provera 2.5 mg, medroxyprogesterone acetate (synthetic progesterone). The study was halted after 5.2 years because of adverse effects. Another study being conducted at the same time using estrogen alone is still in progress and is showing no adverse effects.

The media used figures in their reports that were frightening to women. They reported that women in the study had a 41 percent increase in strokes, a 29 percent increase in heart attacks and doubled rates of blood clots in legs and lungs for women using hormonal therapy. This sounded as if a great number of women had been affected by adverse events in the study. However, when you look behind the headlines into the facts, the numbers were very small. The media reported relative risk increases, (percentage of increase), not absolute chances of risk (actual numbers of increase). Relative risk is the rate of disease in a group exposed to a potential risk factor, divided by the rate of disease in the unexposed group. The actual number from the WHI study were as follows:

Incidence for 10,000 women in one year

	Prempro	Placebo
Heart Attacks	37	30
Strokes	29	21
Breast Cancer	38	30
Blood Clots	34	16
Colorectal Cancer	10 (37% Reduction)	16
Hip Fractures	10 (33% Reduction)	15
Endometrial Cancer	5	6
Overall Deaths	**52**	**53**

As you can see, the adverse events were often counter-balanced by decreases in colon cancer, endometrial cancer and hip fractures. The final death count was **one** less for women who had received HRT.

If you are taking or considering taking HRT and find the study unsettling, consider the final statement by the National Institutes of Health, "This is a relatively small annual increase in risk for an individual woman. Individual women who have participated in the trial and women in the population who have been on progestin should not be unduly alarmed. The results of this study do not apply to estrogens and progestins administered through the transdermal route (patch or medication applied to skin). It remains possible that the transdermal route, which more closely mimics the normal physiology and metabolism, may provide a different risk/benefit profile."

Closer Look at Types of Hormones used in WHI Study

One final fact to consider is that both drugs used in this study were not bio-identical to the hormones found in a woman's body. This study did not compare the plant-based estrogens and progesterone. The estrogen in the study is derived from pregnant horses' urine, with the trade name of Premarin. Premarin stands for Pregnant Mares' Urine (**PRE**gnant **MAR**es' ur**IN**e) and contains 10 - 12 additional hormones not found in the female body. It is often marketed as an organic or a natural product, and it is organic because it comes from a horse. The progestin, Provera, is synthetic progesterone. A company cannot trademark natural plant-based progesterone. They can only trademark it if the delivery system is unique. Thus, drug companies will copy the chemical structure of a compound, making an imitation compound that is synthetic which may respond differently in human use so it can be trademarked. Natural progesterone is needed to maintain pregnancy and the synthetic medroxyprogesterone comes with a warning for miscarriage on the drug label: "The use of medroxyprogesterone during the first four months of pregnancy is not recommended." The synthetic progesterone could promote miscarriage, so there is a vast difference in the two therapies.

National Clinical Guidelines Summary on Study

The Institute for Clinical Systems Improvement (ICSI) which analyzes and recommends best practices in medicine in light of current evidence to healthcare providers, responds to the WHI study with the following guidelines for women. Additional information is listed on the National Guideline Cleaning House web site, www.guideline.gov.

"In light of current data, ICSI and the members of the HRT (hormone replacement therapy) guideline workgroup recommend: The implications of this information do not constitute a medical emergency for women taking HRT and there is no need to stop HRT immediately and no need to see your physician immediately. The risks of HRT for any woman are very low, especially if she has been on HRT for less than five years. The warnings that were publicized apply only to women in the WHI study who were taking Premarin and Provera or a combination pill, Prempro. These warnings do not apply to women taking estrogen alone at this point."

American Cancer Society Study: Overall Survival

American Journal of Epidemiology published a study led by Carmen Rodriguez, Ph.D. and colleagues from the American Cancer Society's Epidemiology and Surveillance Research Department. A group of 290,827 postmenopausal, primarily elderly U.S. women with no history of cancer or cardiovascular disease were enrolled in a prospective study in 1982. After 12 years of followup, death rates from all causes among these women were 12 percent lower among estrogen users compared with non-users.

Types of Estrogen Therapies

Most of the research on hormonal therapy is data from the use of the estrogen Premarin (animal-based). Non-animal based estrogens (plant-based) are more like the normal estrogens made in the female body. These estrogens have a chemical structure that is more like the estrogens women make naturally. Some of the plant-based estrogen replacement therapies now available in the United States are: Alora, Cenestin, Climara, Estrace, Estraderm, Estratab, Estring, FemPatch, Menest, Ogen, Ortho-Est, and Vivelle. They are available in oral form, vaginal suppositories, transdermal cream and transdermal patches applied to the skin.

Compounding pharmacists can customize plant-based therapies to meet the individual needs of a woman. You can locate a compounding pharmacist near you by calling 800-927-4227. Your compounding pharmacist can help you locate a practitioner in your area that specializes in prescribing plant-based hormonal therapies.

The Hormone Decision

The purpose of this chapter was not to make recommendations, but to help women understand the real figures behind the studies rather than the media headlines. Some women have difficulty coping with menopausal symptoms while others do not. Women need to discuss the benefits of hormone replacement with their healthcare provider when approaching menopause if symptoms are troublesome. They also need to discuss the use of the more natural forms of estrogen replacement, using the lowest dose possible to reduce menopausal symptoms, or ask about the many alternative therapies that address menopausal problems.

The benefits and risks vary with individuals and only you and your healthcare provider can make the wisest decision for you. Researchers do not know conclusively, as evidenced by the studies quoted, whether or not women who take HRT have an increased risk of breast cancer over women who do not take HRT, because most of these studies were based on non-human and synthetic hormones often given in higher dosages than they are today. Only when studies become available on today's lower dosages and more natural forms of therapy will we have the answers we need. In the meantime, HRT is a tradeoff between the proven benefits of relieving menopausal symptoms, urinary symptoms and preventing diseases such as osteoporosis and colon cancer versus the possibility of a slight increase in risk for breast cancer. Every woman has to make the decision that is right for her after a discussion about therapy with her own healthcare provider.

Hormone Replacement Therapy After Breast Cancer

In the past several years, the use of estrogen replacement therapy by breast cancer patients after surgery and treatment has gained much attention. This area is controversial, but some healthcare providers are prescribing estrogen replacement after a woman has been disease-free for several years if she is having difficulty with the side effects of menopause. The therapy improves quality of life and some studies show that taking hormones does not promote a recurrence of breast cancer. It appears that the estrogen that affects breast cancer is endogenous (made in your body), not the kind found in supplements. The first choice is usually estrogen cream applied vaginally or Estring, a vaginal ring of estradiol that emits low levels of estradiol for three months, before needing replacement. Estring raises the blood levels of estradiol for a few weeks and then drops to pre-treatment levels, but is very effective in relieving vaginal and urinary symptoms.

Recurrence Study After Estrogen Replacement Therapy

Ellen O'Meara, from the Fred Hutchinson Cancer Research Center and Department of Epidemiology, University of Washington, gathered data from 2755 women who had been diagnosed with invasive breast cancer. The women's ages ranged from 35 to 74 years. They were all enrolled in the same major HMO from 1977 through 1994. Of this group, 174 had received HRT after their breast cancer treatments. Each HRT user was matched to four others of similar age, disease stage, and year of diagnosis who had not been given hormone replacement. As expected, the women who used HRT after diagnosis did show some recurrence. Their rate of breast cancer returning was 17 cases per 1000 women. The blockbuster finding in this report was that women who did not take the HRT had a recurrence rate that was almost double, 30 per 1000. Mortality statistics showed the same pattern. Deaths from breast cancer were five per 1000 person-years in HRT users and 15 per 1000 person-years in nonusers. This means there was three times the risk of dying from breast cancer if estrogen was not taken. Deaths from all causes including heart disease were 16 per 1000 person-years in HRT users and 30 per 1000 person-years in nonusers. So not only did the estrogen protect these women from breast cancer deaths, it also prevented death from other causes.

The authors concluded that these results show that taking estrogen after a breast cancer diagnosis "has no adverse effect on recurrence and mortality." (*Journal of the National Cancer Institute*, Vol. 93, No. 10, 754-761.)

This was the result of one recent study and does not indicate that women should use HRT after a cancer diagnosis; however, it shows that studies are providing data that HRT is not necessarily contraindicated to treat severe menopausal conditions. Ask your healthcare provider for advice about estrogen replacement if you are a breast cancer patient. This is a rapidly evolving area of treatment and the information can change quickly. Your healthcare provider will have the latest information on the use of estrogen replacement after breast cancer. References are listed at the end of this chapter for continuing updates on studies as they become available.

Diet and Lifestyle

Another controversial area is the effect of diet and lifestyle on breast cancer. Lifestyle choices affect health in many ways. High fat diets, regular alcohol use, smoking and exposure to carcinogens (cancer causing substances) have all been studied and may serve as promoters (things that provide an environment for cancer to occur or grow) for breast and other cancers and diseases. Since we don't know what causes breast cancer and no one can point to any one thing and say "this is the cause," the best advice is to select a lifestyle that is identified with overall good health. Follow these lifestyle choices to promote good health:

- Eat a balanced diet of high fiber and low fat foods, and reduce consumption of red meats and animal fats. Fruits, vegetables, and whole grains should compose the major part of your diet.

- Reduce stress to the lowest level possible. Stress has been shown to depress the immune system of the body, allowing an environment where disease is more likely to occur. This may mean that you have to learn to say "no" to some of the demands in your life without feeling guilty.

- Exercise regularly. Exercise reduces stress and helps control weight.

- Monitor alcohol use. Alcoholic beverages consumed on a regular basis have been shown to be a risk factor for breast and other cancers. It is best to keep consumption to an occasional drink, or, if high risk, you may wish to abstain.

- Avoid identified carcinogens such as nitrate-cured foods, pesticides, cigarettes, and various other chemicals.

Dr. Henry Leis, a breast cancer surgeon, advises his patients that:

"A low fat diet is recommended. Other factors of major importance include a high fiber, reduced calorie diet, avoidance of obesity, proper exercise, use of appropriate vitamins and minerals as supplements, limiting consumption of alcohol, salt-cured, smoked and nitrate-cured foods and reducing levels of carcinogens."

Remember:

- All women are at risk for breast cancer. In the last few years, 76 percent of women diagnosed had no family history or other major risk factors.

- Oral contraceptive pills appear to be safe, not increasing the risk of future breast cancer according to recent studies.

- Hormone replacement studies continue to offer conflicting data but HRT seems to be relatively safe if used for a limited period of time to control difficult menopausal symptoms.

- Diet and lifestyle studies also offer conflicting data as to being directly linked to breast cancer, but diet and exercise play an important role in promoting good general health and should be a priority decision in protecting your future health.

Understanding the Role of Reproductive Hormones

A woman's hormones play a large part in her reproductive cycle. The levels vary almost daily. These hormonal changes affect the breast and the uterus. Most women are more aware of hormonal changes because of their menstrual cycle and the potential for pregnancy. However, while the uterus is undergoing changes the breast is also busy preparing for pregnancy.

Hormonal Changes in Menstrual Cycle:

Changing levels of hormones cause a woman's body to prepare her uterus for pregnancy. Most menstrual periods have a 28-day cycle, with the beginning of the menstrual flow usually considered day one. During the menstrual flow and for several days after, the hormones estrogen and progesterone are low. At the same time the follicle-stimulating hormone (FHS) and luteinizing hormone (LH) are higher, sending a message to the ovaries to develop an egg (oocyte). (See chart on next page.)

Day 1 Menstrual flow begins.

Day 6 One oocyte is ready. This oocyte starts making estrogen, which rebuilds the lining of the uterus.

Day 12 LH and FSH cause the follicle (the corpus luteum, a sac in which egg matures) to rupture.

Day 14 The egg is released (ovulation) and the corpus luteum now makes high levels of progesterone to maintain the uterine lining. The egg travels down the tubes as it waits to be fertilized.

Day 28 If the egg is not fertilized the corpus luteum degenerates and the levels of estrogen and progesterone drop greatly. This causes the lining of the uterus to shed and the menstrual bleeding to begin.

Breast Changes:

Hormones cause acini (fluid producing cells) to increase fluid production and stores 3 - 6 teaspoons of fluid in each breast before a menstrual period causing the breasts to feel tender and enlarged. If pregnancy does not occur, hormonal levels plummet, and the breasts have to reabsorb fluid.

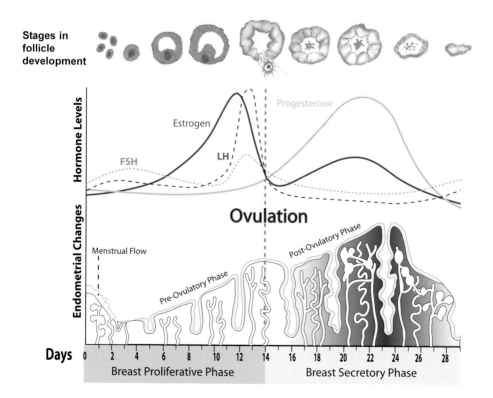

Resources for Diet and Hormonal Issues in Breast Health

If you have questions about diet or hormones in breast health, you may contact the following organizations for information on current trends and studies.

American Cancer Society
1599 Clifton Road, NE
Atlanta, GA 30329-4151
1-800-ACS-2345
www.cancer.org

Hormone Foundation
8401 Connecticut Avenue, Suite 900
Chevy Chase, MD 20815-5817
1-800-HORMONE
www.hormone.org

National Menopause Society
Post Office Box 94527
Cleveland, Ohio 44101
440-442-7550
www.menopause.org

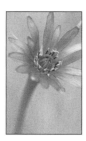

CHAPTER 11

I'M HIGH RISK: WHAT DO I DO?

If you have a family history of breast cancer on your mother's or father's side, you are considered **high risk** for the disease. High risk is a term that terrorizes thousands of women each year after a family member's diagnosis of breast cancer. Thoughts of "this can happen to me, too" can cloud your future and fill you with fear. Often this fear may be so overwhelming that some women avoid taking necessary precautionary measures while others become super-zealous and obsessive in checking their breasts. What is a normal, healthy and balanced approach to breast care if you are considered high risk?

In some ways, being considered high risk may be a blessing—one that could save your life. You may wonder how. Because of a family member's breast cancer, you and your healthcare provider will watch your breasts and health more carefully. If cancer should occur, close monitoring should find it in an early stage when it is most treatable. Women with no history may lack the motivation to be diligent and may ignore guidelines for early detection and screening, resulting in late detection. Don't be frightened of the term "high risk."

High risk does **not** mean that you will get cancer. It is, however, like a yellow light, a warning to be cautious. A family history is no reason for panic; rather, it should be motivation to learn steps for protection and early detection. Based on current information, approximately seven percent of breast cancer patients have a family history of having a mutated gene that places them in a very high-risk category.

If your family member's breast cancer was diagnosed after menopause, first degree relatives (mother, sister, father, brother) are at two to three times greater risk for having breast cancer. If the cancer occurred before menopause or if cancer was found in both breasts, the risk increases approximately five times. Breast cancer that occurs before menopause or in both breasts seems to have a higher incidence of being genetically inherited. It is important for you to know the type of cancer your mother, father, sister, brother, or close relative had and to provide this information to your healthcare provider. (Male breast cancer in the family is now included as a risk factor.)

Components for a Healthy Lifestyle if You Are High Risk

■ Find a healthcare provider who understands your risk and takes a special interest in early detection for breast cancer. Look for a healthcare provider whom you feel comfortable talking with about your breasts and who supports you in learning how to monitor your breasts.

■ Provide your healthcare provider with the name of the type of breast cancer your relative had (there are approximately 15 different major types of breast cancer with variations in how they are found and treated). Breast cancer that is hereditary may show up in the same manner as the relative's cancer; therefore, knowing this is helpful for early detection. For example, if your sister's cancer did not show up on a mammogram, your healthcare provider should not depend on a mammogram alone to detect potential problems.

■ Learn how to perform a breast self-exam from a qualified person.

■ Perform a breast self-exam during the **same time** of your monthly cycle. Allow time to perform a thorough exam. **Do not examine your breasts more than once a month**. This is not necessary. Because the breasts are changing during the month, random checking could cause confusion about what is normal for your breasts.

■ Mammography screening guidelines for high-risk women vary. Most agree that if there is a family history, yearly mammography with a baseline at 35 years is important. If the family history includes a pre-menopausal breast cancer, mammography starting ten years earlier than when the relative's breast cancer occurred is often a recommended guideline.

Monitor those lifestyle factors that have been implicated as risk factors. The following changes in lifestyle have proven to promote better general health and decrease the risk of many other diseases.

■ Avoid high fat diets, especially animal fats. A low-fat, high-fiber diet is a wise choice. Replace sugary, fatty foods with a diet of fresh fruit, vegetables and whole grains.

- Monitor alcohol consumption. Alcohol consumption has been proven to promote breast cancer and other diseases. Drink in moderation—or better yet, not at all. Remember, beer and wine are alcoholic beverages.

- Avoid carcinogens (proven cancer-causing agents) that have been identified in many food additives and chemicals in the environment.

- Check with your healthcare provider regarding vitamin and mineral supplements. Some studies have shown that antioxidant vitamins and minerals (A, C, E, Selenium) may help eliminate free radicals (harmful molecules that can cause cellular damage) from your body.

- Stay active. Exercise reduces stress. Stress has been shown to have a direct effect on the immune system by lowering its ability to fight disease. Start a walking program or join an exercise group.

- Address your anxiety about being high risk. Talk to a professional about your fears. Breast health educators are located in most comprehensive breast centers. Support groups are available in some areas for women having family members with breast cancer. Support groups foster positive steps of action against misinformation and help you evaluate the latest information on fighting the disease.

- After a relative's diagnosis of breast cancer, it is time to face the fear of being high risk and plan to take steps of action. Lifestyle changes, along with early detection and screening, should assure that if cancer occurs, it will be found early, when it can be treated most successfully.

Remember, high risk is not a diagnosis, only a caution light.

Ductal Lavage

Ductal lavage is a new procedure recommended only for women who are at high risk for breast cancer. The procedure collects cells from inside one or several ducts of the milk ductal system (where most breast cancers begin), or at an area that produces a discharge. Ductal lavage is performed in a doctor's office or in an outpatient facility.

Procedure for Ductal Lavage:
1. The nipple area may be scrubbed to remove the small keratin plugs of the nipple openings. An anesthetic cream is applied to numb the nipple area. A suction device is placed over the nipple to gently draw drops of fluid from the nipple duct openings. The fluid droplets help locate the milk ducts' openings on the surface of the nipple for the procedure.

95

2. A small catheter (tube) is inserted into a milk duct opening on the nipple. A small amount of anesthetic is infused into the duct to numb the inside.

3. Saline (salt) water is injected through the catheter to irrigate the duct. The fluid is then aspirated back into a syringe to collect the fluid and cells from the breast duct.

4. The fluid is sent to a pathology laboratory for a cytopathological examination of the cells. By observing changes in the normal cells that line the ducts, a physician can determine if the cells examined put a woman at higher risk for breast cancer.

Ductal lavage is considered appropriate only for women who are at high risk for breast cancer. Ductal lavage has detected a few early stage malignancies, however, and research is currently underway to determine if the procedure is reliable as a predictor of breast cancer. Because the breast has 6 - 10 duct openings, and only one or two ducts are evaluated from one or both breasts, the procedure has limitations as a complete evaluation of the entire breast ductal system.

Inherited Breast Cancer Genes

In 1994 and 1995 two genes were identified that are directly related to breast and ovarian cancer. The genes, BRCA1 and BRCA2 (BR = breast, CA = cancer), are directly related to the potential to have breast or ovarian cancer.

Current data reports that 7 percent of breast cancers and 10 percent of ovarian cancers are associated with an inheritance of one of these mutated genes. Our genes contain the blueprint for features inherited from our parents. Everyone has two copies of all the genes in their body. One comes from their father, and one from their mother. In most people, these genes function normally, but in some individuals, one copy of these genes carries a mutation (alteration from normal). So a father's family history of cancer is equally important to evaluate the risk for either of these breast cancer-related genes. These mutations cause a loss in the ability of the genes to repair damage that occurs during one's lifetime. In other words, you inherit one gene that does not function properly—it is defective. Inherited mutations in these genes greatly increase the probability of a carrier to have breast or ovarian cancer in their lifetime. If a mother or father carried the mutated gene, there is a 50 percent chance that you did not inherit the gene.

Estimated Lifetime Risk

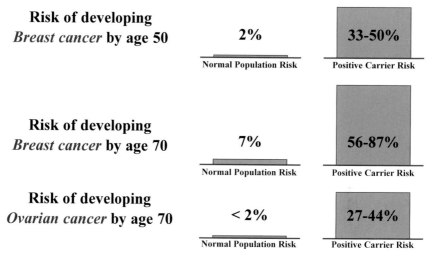

Risk of developing
Breast cancer **by age 50**   2%   33-50%

Normal Population Risk   Positive Carrier Risk

Risk of developing
Breast cancer **by age 70**   7%   56-87%

Normal Population Risk   Positive Carrier Risk

Risk of developing
Ovarian cancer **by age 70**   < 2%   27-44%

Normal Population Risk   Positive Carrier Risk

If you have a family history of breast or ovarian cancer, talk to a healthcare professional about your potential to have inherited one of these genes. They will evaluate your family history for several generations and all types of cancer to determine if you are a candidate for genetic testing.

Testing for inherited BRCA1 or BRCA2 gene mutations is indicated for:

- Individuals with a personal or family history of breast cancer before age 50 or ovarian cancer at any age

- Individuals with two or more primary diagnoses of breast and/or ovarian cancer

- Individuals of Ashkenazi Jewish descent with a personal or family history of breast cancer before age of 50 or ovarian cancer at any age

- Male breast cancer patients

It is highly advised that before testing you talk to a counselor about the benefits and possible psychological impact of testing. Testing is simply done by drawing a vial of blood from you. The testing provides even more helpful information if blood is also drawn from the family member who has had breast or ovarian cancer. Using the cancer patient's blood allows the test to determine if their cancer was caused by an inherited mutation. If positive, other family members can then be tested for the same mutation. The collected blood sample is sent to a specialized lab where extensive evaluation of these two genes is performed to see if cell mutations are present. Because these mutations are inherited, the mutation in the genes can be found in any tissue from your body. Therefore, blood can be used to identify the genes.

If your test is negative, you will then be considered for breast surveillance as recommended by your healthcare provider. If your test comes back positive for one of the genes, you have choices to make in collaboration with your healthcare provider on your breast and ovary surveillance. Choices range from closer screening surveillance to prophylactic surgery.

Recommend Surveillance of Women with Positive Mutations

- Monthly self-exam starting at age 18 - 21 and annual or semiannual clinical exams starting at 25
- Yearly mammography beginning at age 25 - 35
- Annual or semiannual transvaginal ultrasound and blood testing for elevations in CA-125 to detect ovarian cancer beginning at age 25 - 35

Chemoprevention (medications for prevention)

- Tamoxifen for breast cancer
- Oral contraceptives to reduce ovarian cancer

Surgery

- Prophylactic bilateral mastectomy to reduce the risk of breast cancer by 90 percent
- Prophylactic bilateral removal of ovaries to reduce the risk of ovarian cancer by 96 percent

Genetic testing has opened a new opportunity for many women with a significant family history of breast cancer or ovarian cancer to determine if they are truly high risk. This testing is the best way to determine if you are actually at increased risk for breast cancer or if you are at the general population's risk for breast cancer according to your age.

If you would like more information on risk evaluation or to locate a center near you to talk to about your risk, Myriad Genetic Laboratories has professional educators to guide you to local resources. Call Myriad at 1-800-469-7423 or visit them on their web site at: www.myriadtests.com.

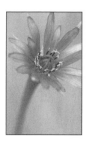

CHAPTER 12

WHEN DISEASE HAS BEEN RULED OUT: THE CAFFEINE CONNECTION

Caffeine has long been debated as a contributor to breast pain and lumpiness connected with fibrocystic changes. Some studies agree and some do not. What we do know is that some women have reported relief by changing their caffeine intake. And the good news is that changing these patterns does not require prescriptions and costly interventions. It is something that you can try for yourself and evaluate. After you have consulted with a healthcare provider, if disease has been ruled out, a caffeine-free diet may be recommended to reduce your pain or lumpiness associated with fibrocystic changes. Some women have found that their breasts are very sensitive to caffeine products and that a diet lower in caffeine significantly reduces the amount of breast discomfort they experience. The following information will help you understand how to best manage the caffeine reduction in your diet.

Reducing caffeine in your diet may cause you to experience headaches. Therefore, it may help to **reduce your intake gradually**. For example, if you are drinking four cups of coffee a day, reduce the amount to three cups the first several days and then to two cups. Gradual reduction will minimize headaches. If you decide to eliminate caffeine completely (going cold turkey), headaches may last from one to seven days. This is a normal reaction.

After you go on a caffeine-free diet, it will take approximately two months to show an improvement in the discomfort and pain associated with fibrocystic changes. Some women respond more slowly and may not see a change for up to a year; others report improvement in weeks. Still others find no relief from reduced caffeine.

Most people associate caffeine with coffee consumption. However, there are many products that contain high amounts of caffeine. Intake of these products also needs to be reduced or eliminated. Read carefully the labels of products to check for caffeine amounts. Listed below are some commonly used products and the approximate amount of caffeine they contain.

Caffeine Containing Products

Product	Caffeine Milligrams
Coffee:	
Drip (5 oz.)	146
Percolated (5 oz.)	110
Instant, regular (5 oz.)	53
Decaffeinated brewed (5 oz.)	3
Decaffeinated instant (5 oz.)	2
Tea:	
Brewed (5 oz.)	60-75
Instant (5 oz.)	30
Iced tea, canned (12 oz.)	22-36
Cocoa & Chocolate:	
Cocoa (water mix) (6 oz.)	10
Baking Chocolate (1 oz.)	6
Chocolate bar (2-3 oz.)	10
Soft Drinks (12 oz.):	
Mountain Dew	52
Mello Yellow	52
Tab	52
Coke Classic	46
Diet Coke	46
Sunkist Orange	42
Shasta Cola	42
Diet Mr. Pibb	40
Mr. Pibb	40
Dr. Pepper	38
Diet Dr. Pepper	37
Pepsi Cola	37

Product	Caffeine Milligrams
Soft Drinks (12 oz.):	
Royal Crown Cola	36
Diet-Rite Cola	34
Diet Pepsi	34
Diet Mello Yellow	12
7-Up	0
Sierra Mist	0
Sprite	0
Minute Maid Orange	0
Diet 7-Up	0
Diet Sunkist Orange	0
Diet Sierra Mist	0
Fanta Orange	0
Fresca	0
Hires Root Beer	0

Non-Prescription Drugs	Caffeine Milligrams
Stimulants-standard dose:	
No-Doz	200
Vivarin	200
Pain Relievers-standard dose:	
Excedrin (2 tablets)	130
Anacin (2 tablets)	64
Midol (2 tablets)	65
Goody's Powder (1 powder)	32
BC Powder (1 powder)	32
Plain aspirin (any brand)	0
Cold Remedies:	
Dristan	32
Coryban-D	30

Herbal Products Similar to Caffeine

Some herbal supplements have been identified as having a substance identical to caffeine, called guaranine. Guarana (contains 4 percent guaranine) or Kola Nut has the same effect as caffeine on the body. Recognizing these names may help you identify supplements that could trigger a reaction similar to caffeine.

Remember:

- Read the labels of all products for their contents. This chapter includes just a partial listing of many commonly used products that contain caffeine.

- Caffeine reduction has helped some women with breast tenderness and pain. However, it may take several months or longer to evaluate the effectiveness.

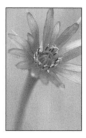

CHAPTER 13

THE CHALLENGE OF MONITORING YOUR BREASTS

One of the ways to protect your breast health is to monitor your breasts by learning breast self-exam (refer to Chapter 14). Remember, it is normal to have lumpy breasts. Learn your normal pattern of lumpiness and report any change to your healthcare provider. With clinical exams by a healthcare provider and screening mammograms at the recommended intervals, you can be assured that you are using the most effective methods of detection for breast cancer. If cancer does occur, it may be found early when it can be treated most successfully. Become partners with your healthcare provider in monitoring your breast health. Remember, if you do find a lump or a change, 80 percent of such findings turn out to be benign changes that are not life threatening.

- **Learn how to perform a breast self-exam**

- **Have a clinical exam as part of a regular health exam and shortly before a mammogram**

- **Have a mammogram on the recommended basis:**

    35 - 40   **Optional; baseline screening**

    40 - up   **Every year**

    High risk women   **Healthcare provider's recommendation**

    Anytime with a suspicious finding

Your efforts are very valuable in protecting your health and future against breast cancer. Your healthcare provider needs you as a partner to monitor for changes and report them if they occur.

Tips For Having Your Mammogram

- Schedule your mammogram at the end of your menstrual period. If you are menopausal and cycle off of supplemental estrogen, schedule your exam for the day you resume your medication. This scheduling reduces the discomfort from compression of the paddles during the mammogram.

- Do not wear deodorant, perfume, or powders on your upper body to the exam. They may show up as artifacts (unusual findings) on the film. Wear a skirt, shorts, or pants so that you will only have to remove your shirt for the exam. A gown will be provided and only the technologist who positions you will be present for the mammogram.

- If a past mammogram was uncomfortable, discuss this with your mammographer. However, compression, though uncomfortable for a few seconds, is necessary to ensure the best picture possible.

- Some women have found that discomfort is less if they reduce the amount of caffeine they consume for several days before the exam, or if they take ibuprofen for several days prior.

- Select a facility that has a Food and Drug Administration (FDA) certification to ensure that you are receiving the highest quality mammogram possible. This certification is awarded to the facility if the equipment, procedures, mammography technologists and radiologists meet the FDA's standards of care. A certificate will be displayed in the facility. Ask your provider if you do not see one.

- Ask your technologist or radiologist to discuss questions you may have about your particular breast problems. They are your partners in monitoring your breasts and helping you find answers to your problems.

- If you change mammography centers, ask your previous provider for your old mammogram(s) to take with you. Your radiologist will compare your old mammogram with your new one.

CHAPTER 14

BREAST SELF-EXAM

Breast self-exam (BSE) has often been a controversial topic. The goal of BSE is not to look for cancer but to learn your own breasts well enough to recognize a change that would need evaluation by a healthcare provider. Cancer cannot be diagnosed by anyone's fingers; this takes screening tests and a biopsy. The goal of an exam is to identify those changes if they should occur and to work as a partner with your healthcare provider in protecting your breast health.

Interesting Facts About Breast Self-Exam

- Breast self-exam (BSE) is the an effective way to find a lump that can be felt. Women find approximately 90 percent of all lumps and then consult a physician.

- Breast self-exam is the most cost-effective way to monitor your breasts—it's free! It only takes about 15 minutes per exam.

- 80 percent of all lumps biopsied are not cancer.

- Breast self-exam can find some cancers that do not show up on a mammogram.

- 50 percent of all lumps are found in the axillary tail (the quarter of the breast from the nipple to the underarm area).

Tips For Breast Self-Exam

- To become proficient, learn BSE from a professional—your physician or a trained healthcare provider.

- Perform a **BSE** during the same time in each of your monthly cycles. **Caution**—women who examine their breasts at different times in their cycles or more than once a month may become confused because of all the normal changes the breasts undergo.

- Set aside a quiet, uninterrupted time to perform your exam. Turn off the television and radio. Do not answer the phone. Concentration allows you to remember what is normal in your breasts and to detect early changes.

- Exams performed in the shower are not the best method of surveillance and are not recommended as the best method of breast self-exam.

A New Improved Method Of Breast Self-Exam

The **MammaCare®** method described in the following section is a modification of the traditional breast self-exam developed as a result of a study at the University of Florida and funded by the National Cancer Institute. These modifications are now considered state-of-the-art in breast self-exam methods.

Changes in the position for the exam, areas to check, hand positions, pressures to use and checking for lymph node changes may be new to you. These changes came from MammaCare's® extensive research to determine what would help a woman find changes in her breast at an early stage. Read through the instructions and look at the drawings. You will first read an explanation and see an illustration of the changes. Then there will be instructions on how to use these changes in your breast self-exam.

Position For Exam: Side-lying Position

1. Lie on the side opposite of the breast you are to examine and pull your knees up slightly.

2. Rotate the shoulder of the breast you are examining to the flat of the bed. You will examine your right breast with your left hand and your left breast with your right hand. You may place a small pillow against the middle of your back to keep you in a side-lying position. It is important to keep your hips rotated. Your nipple should point toward the ceiling. This side-lying position allows you to examine most effectively the outer half of your breast by keeping the tissues spread out evenly. If you are examining your right breast, place your right hand on your **forehead** with your palm up. This is **very important**.

3. Keep this position as you examine your breast with the opposite hand until you reach your nipple. Then **rotate** your **hips** to lie flat on the bed and complete your exam **flat on your back**. Remove your hand from your forehead and place it on the bed. This allows the inner part of the breast to be spread thin on the chest wall.

Side-Lying Position

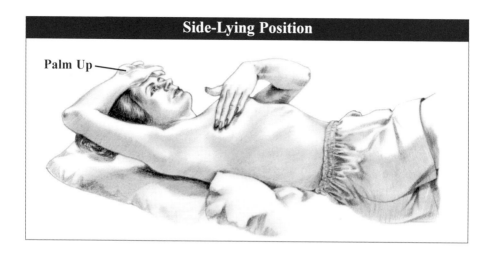

Palm Up

Fifty percent of all cancers occur in the upper, outer quarter of the breast, called the **axillary tail**. The side-lying position with your hand placed palm up on your forehead allows you to examine this tissue thoroughly. Take extra time during your exam in this area.

Axillary Tail

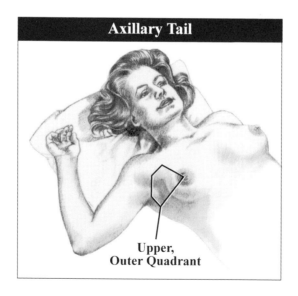

Upper,
Outer Quadrant

Perimeters: Area You Examine

- Middle notch of the collarbone, following under collarbone until you reach the middle of your underarm
- Down from the middle underarm area to the bra line
- Follow the bra line across until you reach the middle of the breastbone
- Follow from the middle of the breastbone back up to the collarbone notch.

The reason for the larger boundaries is that the breast gland is a large gland that covers most of this area, not just the breast mound.

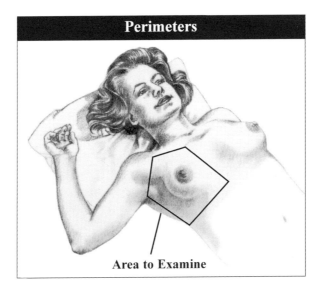

Perimeters

Area to Examine

Palpation: Finger Positions

1. Use the flat pads of your three middle fingers, from the first joint down to the fingertips. Do not use the tips of your fingers.

2. Place your hand in a flat, bowing position on your breast. Your smallest finger will automatically extend upward when you have the correct flat, bowing position for your hand for the exam. (See the illustration on the next page.)

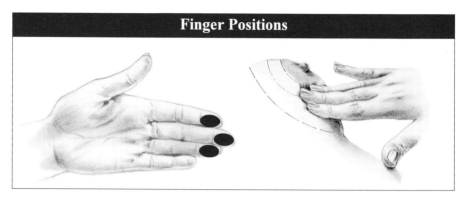

Pressures: Three Levels

Three levels of pressure will be used to make three small, dime-size circles on your breast tissue:

1. **Light pressure**—barely moves the top layer of skin

2. **Medium pressure**—goes halfway through the thickness of the breast tissue

3. **Deep pressure**—goes to the base of the breast

Do not lift your hand or release the pressure on your breast as you make the three circles. Pressure will not injure your breasts and is not painful. By using varying pressures, you examine the full thickness of the breasts and reduce the possibility of displacing small lumps into fibrous tissues or your rib area.

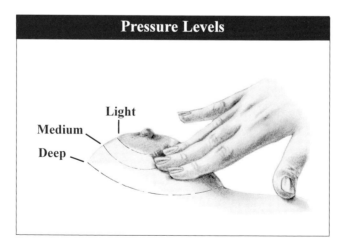

Pattern of Exam: Parallel Vertical Strips

■ Begin your exam under the arm and make rows of straight lines up and down on the breast tissue, like the pattern people use to mow grass or vacuum a carpet.

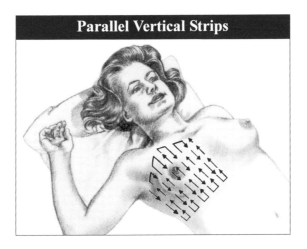

Parallel Vertical Strips

Practice: Examining Your Breast

1. Assume the side-lying position described earlier with your hand on your forehead **palm up**.

2. Begin in the area of the armpit and make straight rows of circles using three pressures in each spot, not releasing pressure as you spiral downward; be sure **not** to miss any tissue.

3. When you reach the nipple, roll over flat on your back and place your hand on the bed at a right angle.

4. **Do not squeeze the nipple**; examine the nipple area using the same method with three levels of pressure. Report any discharge not associated with the onset of a menstrual period, hormonal usage, sexual stimulation, or excessive manipulation of the breasts. A bloody discharge or a discharge from only one breast needs to be reported promptly.

5. When one side is completed, repeat the method for the opposite breast.

6. Check the **lymph nodes** under the collarbone, over the collarbone and under the arm. These areas are shown in the following figure. Enlarged nodes feel distinctively firmer than surrounding tissues, like a small pea. Report any enlargement found. Infection may also cause enlarged lymph nodes.

Check the Lymph Nodes

Lymph Nodes

Visual Exam Positions

Visually examine your breasts in front of a mirror, using four different arm positions. Because some cancers never form a hard lump, visual inspection to observe changes is necessary. Stand in front of a mirror and look closely at your breasts in the positions illustrated on the next page, as you turn from side to side.

In each position, look at your breasts for changes in the following:

1. **Shape of the breast**, including the shape of the areola and the nipple. Compare one breast to the other. One breast may normally be larger than the other, but changes in size should not occur suddenly. One breast may also sit higher on the chest wall.

2. **Skin**—for any **rash, redness, orange peel skin, dimpling** (pulling in), **bulging out, moles,** or any type of a **sore** or **bump**.

3. **Nipple**—for any **crusty material** caused by a discharge, **rash** around the nipple, or **inversion** (pulling in) of the nipple.

4. **Vein pattern on the chest**—for a noticeable increase in the **number or size of veins** in one breast compared to the other.

Arms at Side	Raised Above Head
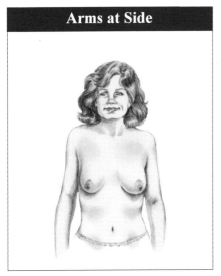	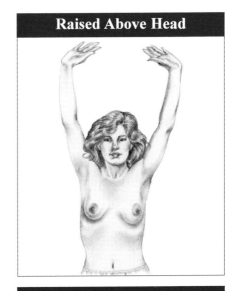

Bending Forward	Hands on Hips Pressing Down
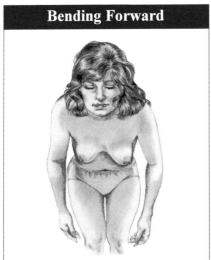	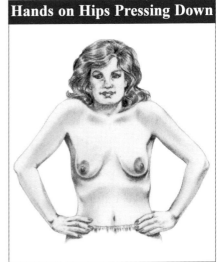

Remember:

■ A breast self-exam is not an event that any woman looks forward to preforming. However, it is an important component of good health practices, like flossing your teeth. After you complete your exam, congratulate yourself for taking an active part in your breast health care.

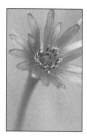

CHAPTER 15

BREAST EXAM AFTER BREAST CANCER SURGERY

If you have had surgery for breast cancer, you will need to continue to perform a breast self-exam. Recommendations for starting exams after breast surgery are as follows:

■ **Lumpectomy patients** should begin breast self-exam at the completion of radiation therapy or when the incision has healed completely.

■ **Mastectomy patients** should begin examination of the surgical site approximately two to three months after surgery. You should carefully examine the scar and the entire chest wall area on the side of the mastectomy.

■ **Reconstructive surgery patients** should examine the entire reconstruction area beginning when their incision is completely healed, approximately two to three months after surgery. Bilateral reconstruction patients should carefully examine the skin, underarm areas and lymph nodes above the collarbone.

Normal Changes In Surgical Area

There are some normal changes you will need to be aware of during your exam of your lumpectomy breast or the scar area of a mastectomy.

■ Pain in the surgical breast that is sporadic, with a shooting sensation from the incision, is not uncommon (especially after a lumpectomy). This pain can occur for months.

■ Incision scars may have areas that feel firm to touch. This is caused by scar tissue formation during healing. Areas where drains were inserted may also feel firm. This is normal. Becoming familiar with these changes soon after your surgery will prevent misinterpretation of these normal post-surgical changes. Very rarely does cancer recur in the incisional area the first few months after surgery.

Changes in the Radiated Breast:

- Darkening in color of the area (suntanned appearance)
- Edema (swelling of the breast tissues for up to a year)
- Gradual decrease in swelling
- Slight decrease in size when edema subsides
- Firmness of the radiated tissues, often feeling lumpy
- Skin thickening (greatest in the area of the nipple and areola following a lumpectomy)
- Decreased sensitivity

It is helpful to become familiar with the normal changes occurring after radiation therapy. Because of the sensitivity of the radiated breast or incisional scar area, some women feel that applying powder or hand lotion to their hands prior to their self-exam assists in moving their hands freely over the breast tissue.

Suggestions For Breast Self-Exam After Surgery

After breast surgery, it is normal for you to approach the idea of breast self-exam with anxiety. Some women feel overwhelmed at the idea of monitoring their surgical area and remaining breast. If you have experienced these feelings, you are normal. One of the best methods to reduce this anxiety is to begin your exams by having a healthcare provider examine your breast(s) and talk to you about the changes they find during their exam. With assurance that there is no evidence of an abnormality in your breast(s), you can begin your exam knowing that what you feel is normal. Very seldom does a recurrence happen in the surgical breast months after surgery.

Some women may continue to feel that they cannot psychologically handle the task of monitoring their breasts with self-exams. If you feel this way, discuss this with your physician. This feeling is not uncommon and is not a sign of weakness on your part. Your physician will talk with you about a plan of surveillance to monitor your breasts. Some healthcare providers offer the services of a qualified nurse for the exams, or they may have you return more frequently to see them. The goal is to have your breast(s) monitored; it does not require that you be the examiner if this creates too much anxiety.

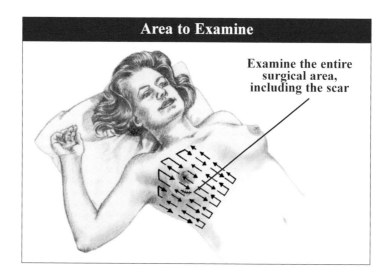

Area to Examine

Examine the entire surgical area, including the scar

Mammograms After Surgery

It is very important to continue to have your breast(s) monitored after breast cancer surgery. Ask your physician what schedule is recommended and follow this guideline. Some physicians recommend more frequent mammograms the first few years after breast conservation surgery. Lumpectomy patients may be asked to have a mammogram every six months the first two years after their surgery and annually thereafter. Occasionally, a physician may recommend a mammogram on the mastectomy site of the remaining skin and muscle.

Remind your physician if your annual checkup does not include a mammogram. Remember to schedule your mammogram when your breast(s) is least tender, usually at the end of your menstrual period if you are pre-menopausal.

If you had reconstructive surgery with implants, be sure that the technologist is experienced in performing mammograms on breasts with implants. Ask your reconstructive surgeon for recommendations for a facility and technologist to perform your exam.

Breast Self-Exam After Surgery

Examine the entire breast and surgical area. Carefully examine lymph node areas. Report any areas that are firm, feeling like a small, soft pea.

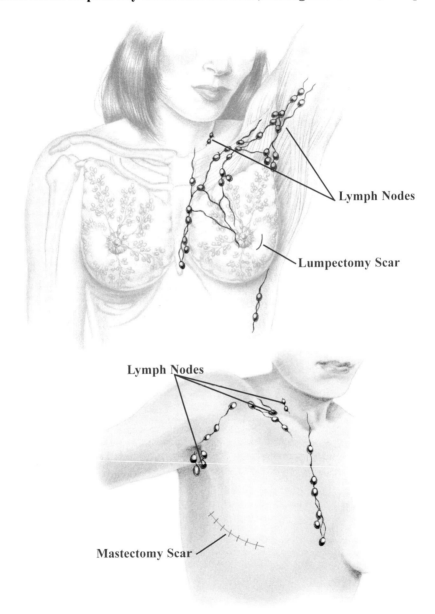

Lymph Nodes

Lumpectomy Scar

Lymph Nodes

Mastectomy Scar

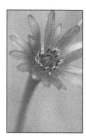

CHAPTER 16

THE DRUG CONNECTION AND BREAST PROBLEMS

One of the **most common causes** of breast tenderness, breast pain, breast discharge and changes in the size of the breasts are over-the-counter and prescription **medications**. Many medications can cause changes that are often mistaken for problems originating in the breasts. Because drugs can produce different responses in different women, some women may experience side effects from a medication, while others have no response.

The categories of drugs that may cause breast changes are hormonal, blood pressure, heart, pain relievers, antibiotics, antidepressants and gastrointestinal medications. When you review the following lists, you may find that you are taking more than one drug that can cause breast changes, increasing your potential for problems.

If you are experiencing a change in your breasts and are presently taking any of the listed medications, you may want to discuss this with your health-care provider. **Do not stop taking any prescribed medication without consulting your healthcare provider.** However, you may decide to stop taking over-the-counter medications to evaluate your breasts' response. Most healthcare providers recommend four to six weeks without medication to determine whether a medication is the cause.

The PDR® *(Physician's Desk Reference) Guide to Drug Interactions, Side Effects, Indications*™ lists the drugs that may affect the breasts. Pharmaceutical manufacturers supply Medical Economics, the publisher, with the information provided in the PDR®. Companies describe known side effects of their medications using different terminology for what may be the same breast changes.

To be precise in reporting, the PDR® and this book have used the manufacturers' specific wording in reporting possible side effects of their medications (* denotes a manufacturer's term) for the subcategories. All the drugs listed may cause or exacerbate breast changes and are listed by their trade names under major categories of change.

117

General Breast Changes

Unspecified* Breast Changes
Brevicon
Demulen
Desogen Tablets
Emcyt Capsules (10-66%)
Loestrin
Lo/Ovral Tablets
Lo/Ovral-28 Tablets
Lupron Depot-PED (Less than 2%)
Micronor Tablets
Modicon
Nordette-21 Tablets
Nordette-28 Tablets
Norinyl
Nor-Q-D Tablets
Ortho-Cept Tablets
Ortho-Cyclen Tablets
Ortho-Novum
Ortho-Tri-Cyclen
Ovral Tablets
Ovral-28 Tablets
Ovrette Tablets
Proglycem
Rogaine Topical Solution
Tri-Norinyl
Triphasil-21 Tablets
Triphasil-28 Tablets

Breast Size Changes

Unspecified*
Depo-Provera Contraceptive Injection (fewer than 1%)

Breast Atrophy*
Paxil Tablets (Rare)
Zoladex (33%)

Breast Size Reduction*
Danocrine Capsules
Supprelin Injection (2-3%)
Synarel Nasal Solution (10%)

Breast Engorgement*
Adalat CC (Less than 1%)
Anafranil Capsules (Rare)
Betaseron for SC Injection
Desyrel and Desyrel Dividose
Effexor (Rare)
Haldol Decanoate
Haldol Injection, Tablets and Concentrate
Mellaril
Permax Tablets (Rare)
Ser-Ap-Es Tablets
Synarel Nasal Solution (Less than 1%)
Zoladex (Greater than 1% but less than 5%)

Enlargement*
Adapin Capsules
Aldoclor Tablets
Aldomet Ester HCI Injection
Aldomet Oral
Aldoril Tablets
Anafranil Capsules (Up to 2%)
Asendin Tablets (Less than 1%)
Brevicon
Claritin (2% or fewer)
Demser Capsules (Infrequent)
Demulen
Depakene
Depakote
Desogen Tablets
Desyrel and Desyrel Dividose
Diethylstilbestrol Tablets
Effexor (Rare)
Elavil

Enlargement (continued)*
Emcyt Capsules (60%)
Endep Tablets
Estrace Cream and Tablets
Estraderm Transdermal System
Estradurin
Estratab Tablets
Estratest
Etrafon
Flexeril Tablets (Rare)
Indocin Capsules (Less than 1%)
Indocin I.V. (Less than 1%)
Indocin (Less than 1%)
Levlen/Tri-Levlen
Limbitrol
Loestrin
Ludiomil Tablets (Isolated reports)
Menest Tablets
Micronor Tablets
Modicon
Navane Capsules and Concentrate
Navane Intramuscular
Norinyl
Norpramin Tablets
Nor-Q D Tablets
Ogen Tablets
Ogen Vaginal Cream
Ortho-Cept Tablets
Ortho-Cyclen Tablets
Ortho Dienestrol Cream
Ortho-Est
Ortho-Novum
Ortho-Tri-Cyclen Tablets
Ovcon
PMB 200 and PMB 400
Pamelor
Premarin Intravenous
Premarin with Methyltestosterone

Premarin Tablets
Premarin Vaginal Cream
Proscar Tablets
ProSom Tablets (Rare)
Prozac Pulvules & Liquid, Oral Solution (Rare)
Sinequan
Stilphostrol Tablets and Ampules
Supprelin Injection (1-10%)
Surmontil Capsules
Synarel Nasal Solution for Central Precocious Puberty
Thorazine
Thyrel TRH (a small number)
Tofranil Ampules
Tofranil Tablets
Tofranil-PM Capsules
Triavil Tablets
Trilafon
Tri-Norinyl
Triphasil-21 Tablets
Triphasil-28 Tablets
Vivactil Tablets
Zoladex (18%)
Zoloft Tablets (Rare)

Gynecomastia *(Enlargement)*
Adalat Capsules (Less than 0.5%)
Adalat C.C. (Rare)
Adapin Capsules
Aldactazide (Not infrequent)
Aldactone (Not infrequent)
Aldoclor
Aldomet Ester HCI Injection
Aldomet Oral
Aldoril Tablets
Anadrol-50 Tablets
Anafranil Capsules (Rare)
Android (Among most common)
Asendin Tablets

Gynecomastia* (continued)

Atromid-S Capsules
Axid Puivules (Rare)
Betaseron for SC Injection
Calan SR Caplets (1% or less)
Calan Tablets (1% or less)
Capoten
Capozide
Catapres Tablets (About 1 in 1000)
Catapres -TTS (Less frequent)
Cipro I.V. (1% or less)
Cipro I.V. Pharmacy Bulk Package
Clinoril Tablets (Rare)
Combipres Tablets (About 1 in 1000)
Compazine
Elavil
Endep Tablets
Etrafon
Eulexin Capsules
Flexeril Tablets (Rare)
Foscavir Injection (1-5%)
Haldol Decanoate
Haldol Injection, Tablets and Concentrate
Halotestin Tablets
IBU (Ibuprofen Tablets, USP)
Indocin Capsules (Less than 1%)
Indocin I.V. (Less than 1%)
INH Tablets
Intron A (Less than 5%)
Isoptin Oral Tablets
Isoptin SR Sustained Release Tablets (1% or less)
Lanoxicaps (Occasional)
Lanoxin Elixir Pediatric
Lanoxin Injection (Occasional)
Lanoxin Injection Pediatric
Lanoxin Tablets (Occasional)
Lescol Capsules
Limbitrol

Loxitane (Rare)
Ludiomil Tablets (Isolated Reports)
Lupron Depot 3.75 mg (Among most frequent)
Lupron Depot 7.5 mg (Less than 5%)
Lupron Depot- PED (Less than 2%)
Lupron Injection (5% or more)
Matulane Capsules
Megace Oral Suspension (1-3%)
Mellaril
Mevacor Tablets (0.5-1%)
Midamor
Moban Tablets and Concentrate
Moduretic
Motrin Tablets
Myerlan Tablets
Navane Capsules and Concentrate
Navane Intramuscular
Nizoral Tablets (Less than 1%)
Norpace
Norpramin
Nydrazid Injection
Oreton Methyl (Among most common)
Orudis Capsules (Rare)
Pamelor
Pepcid Injection (Rare)
Pepcid (Rare)
Pergonal (menotropins for injection, USP)
Pravachol
Pregnyl
Prilosec Delayed-Release Capsules (Less than 1%)
Profasi (chorionic gonadotropin for injection)
Prolixin
Reglan
Rifamate
Sandimmune (1-4%)
Ser-Ap-Es Tablets
Serentil
Sinequan

Gynecomastia (continued)*
Sporanox Capsules (Less than 1%)
Stelazine
Surmontil Capsules
Tagamet
Taractan
Temaril Tablets, Syrup and Spanule (extended-release)
Testoderm Testosterone (Five in 104 patients)
Testred Capsules
Thorazine
Tofranil Ampules
Tofranil-PM Capsules
Tofranil Tablets
Torecan
Trecator-SC Tablets
Triavil Tablets
Trilafon
Vaseretic Tablets
Vasotec I.V.
Vasotec Tablets (0.5%-1%)
Verelan Capsules (Less than 1%)
Vivactil Tablets
Wellbutrin Tablets (Infrequent)
Winstrol Tablets
Wytensin Tablets
Xanax Tablets
Zantac (Occasional)
Zantac Injection and Zantac Injection Premixed
Zocor Tablets
Zoloft Tablets (Rare)
Zyloprim Tablet (Less than 1%)

Breast Lumpiness

*Breast Fibroadenosis**
Ambien Tablets (Rare)
Anafranil Capsules (Rare)
Kerlone Tablets (Less than 2%)

Fibrocystic Breasts*
Betaseron for SC Injection (3%)
Levlen/Tri-Levlen
Micronor Tablets
Modicon
Ortho-Cyclen Tablets
Ortho-Novum
Ortho-Tri-Cyclen Tablets
Permax Tablets (Infrequent)
Prozac Pulvules, Liquid, Oral Solution (Infrequent)

Breast Lumps*
Depo/Provera Contraceptive Injection
Levlen/Tri-Levlen
Ortho-Cyclen Tablets
Ortho-Est
Ortho-Cyclen Tablets

Breast Pain or Tenderness

Breast Pain*
Anafranil (Up to 1%)
Betaseron for SC Injection (7%)
Cardura Tablets (Less than 0.5%)
Clozaril Tablets (Less than 1%)
Cognex Capsules (Infrequent)
Imdur (Less than or equal to 5%)
Lupron Depot 7.5 mg.
Paxil Tablets
Pentasa (Less than 1%)
Procardia XL Extended Release Tablets (Less than 1%)
Prozac Pulvules and Liquid, Oral Solution (Infrequent)
Sporanox Capsules (Less than 1%)
Zoladex (7%)
Zoloft Tablets (Rare)

Breast Tenderness *
Amen Tablets (Rare)
Azactam for Injection (Less than 1%)
Brevicon
Bumex (0.1%)
Cycrin Tablets (Rare)
Demulen (Among most common)
Depo-Provera Contraceptive Injection
Desogen Tablets
Diethylstilbestrol Tablets
Emcyt Capsules (66%)
Estrace Cream and Tablets
Estrace Vaginal Cream
Estraderm Transdermal System
Estratab Tablets
Estratest
Indocin (Less than 1%)
Indocin Capsules
Indocin I.V.
Levlen/Tri-Levlen
Lo/Ovral Tablets
Lo/Ovral-28 Tablets
Loniten Tablets (Less than 1%)
Lupron Depot 7.5 mg.
Lupron Injection (5% or more)
Menest Tablets
Metrodin
Micronor Tablets
Modicon
Norinyl
Norlutate
Nor-Q D Tablets
Ogen Tablets
Ogen Vaginal Cream
Ortho-Cept Tablets
Ortho-Cyclen Tablets
Ortho Dienestrol Cream
Ortho-Est.

Ortho-Novum
Ortho-Tri-Cyclen Tablets
Ovcon Ovral Tablets
Ovral-28 Tablets
Ovrette Tablets
PMB 200 and PMB 400
Premarin Intravenous
Premarin Vaginal Cream
Premarin with Methyltestosterone
Premarin Tablets
Prostin E2 Suppository
Provera Tablets (Rare)
Serophene (clomiphene citrate tablets)
Stilphostrol Tablets and Ampules
Testoderm Testosterone Transdermal System
Levlen/Tri-Levlen
Tri-Norinyl
Triphasil-21 Tablets
Triphasil-28 Tablets
Zoladex (Greater than 1% but less than 5%)

Breast Discharge

*Breast Secretions**
Brevicon
Danocrine Capsules (Rare)
Demulen
Desogen Tablets
Diethylstilbestrol Tablets
Dienestrol Cream
Estratest
Levlen/Tri-Levlen
Loestrin
Menest Tablets
Micronor Tablets
Modicon
Norinyl
Norplant System

Breast Secretions (continued)*
Nor-Q D Tablets
Ogen Vaginal Cream
Ortho-Cept Tablets
Ortho-Cyclen
Ortho Dienestrol Cream
Ortho-Est 0.625 Tablets
Ortho-Est 1.25 Tablets
Ortho-Novum
Ortho-Tri-Cyclen Tablets
Ovcon
PMB 200 and PMB 400
Premarin Intravenous
Premarin Vaginal Cream
Premarin with Methyltestosterone
Stilphostrol Tablets and Ampules
Supprelin Injection
Tri-Norinyl

*Bleeding from the Nipple**
Ceclor Pulvules & Suspension
Depo-Provera Contraceptive Injection (Less than 1%)

*Galactorrhea**
Adapin Capsules
Amen Tablets (Rare)
Asendin Tablets (Less than 1%)
BuSpar (Rare)
Calan SR Caplets (1% or less)
Calan Tablets (1% or less)
Compazine
Cycrin Tablets (Rare)
Demser Capsules (Infrequent)
Depakene Capsules & Syrup
Depakote
Depo-Provera Contraceptive Injection (Fewer than 1%)
Depo-Provera Sterile Aqueous Suspension
Elavil

Endep Tablets
Etrafon
Flexeril Tablets (Rare)
Haldol Decanoate
Haldol Injection, Tablets and Concentrate
Isoptin SR Sustained Release Tablets (1% or less)
Limbitrol
Loxitane (Rare)
Ludiomil Tablets (Isolated reports)
Mellaril
Moban Tablets and Concentrate
Norpramin Tablets
Pamelor
Proglycem
Prolixin Oral Concentrate
Provera Tablets (Rare)
Reglan
Sandostatin Injection (Less than 1%)
Seldane Tablets
Seldane D Extended-ReleaseTablets
Serentil
Sinequan
Stelazine
Surmontil
Tofranil Ampules
Tofranil PM Capsules
Tofranil Tablets
Triavil Tablets
Trilafon
Vivactil Tablets
Xanax Tablets

Remember:

- Women respond differently to medications. Some women will respond with changes in their breasts while others will not.

- If you experience symptoms that cause you concern or have symptoms similar to a malignancy, the cause should be evaluated as soon as possible.

- Most medication-induced breast changes occur in **both** breasts. However, one breast may have more exaggerated symptoms.

- Understanding medications and the changes they may cause in your breasts could save you much anxiety and thousands of dollars in medical costs by avoiding having the problem evaluated with expensive diagnostic tests.

- Often learning the cause of the change in your breasts will make the symptoms much more bearable.

- Stopping some medications may bring relief in days. However, it may take four to six weeks after stopping other medications to evaluate the effect they may have on your breast problem. Times vary because of different medications and different women's responses to them.

- **Do not stop taking any prescription medication without consulting your physician.**

GLOSSARY

It is helpful if you understand the medical terminology used in breast care. A list of the most common medical terms used in breast care follows. If you do not understand the technical language used by healthcare providers, ask them to explain what they mean. This will enable you to be a more effective partner in monitoring your breasts.

A

Abscess - A collection of pus from infection.

Acini - The parts of the breast gland where fluid or milk is produced (singular: acinus).

Acute - Symptoms occurring suddenly, or over a short period of time.

Adenosis Tumor - Benign tumor composed of glands of the breast.

Amenorrhea - Absence of monthly menstrual period.

Analgesic - Medicine given to control pain; for example, aspirin or Tylenol®.

Anesthesia - Medication that causes entire or partial loss of feeling or sensation.

Androgen - A male sex hormone. Androgens may be used in patients with breast disease to treat symptoms of the disease caused from high levels of female hormones.

Areola - The darker, circular area of skin surrounding the nipple.

Aspiration - Procedure of removing fluid or cells from tissue by inserting a needle into the area and drawing the fluid or cells into the syringe.

Asymptomatic - Without obvious signs or symptoms of disease. Cancer may cause symptoms and warning signs; but, especially in its early stages, cancer may develop and grow without producing any symptoms.

Atypical Cells - Cells that are not like normal cells in an area; abnormal. Cancer is the result of atypical cell division.

Atrophy - A decrease in the size of a gland or cells in an area that is benign.

Axilla - The armpit.

Axillary Tail - The portion of the breast extending into the area of the armpit.

Axillary Nodes - The lymph nodes in the axilla (underarm). These are the nodes that are sampled or removed during surgery to see if the cancer has spread beyond the breast. The number of nodes in this area varies in different women.

B

Benign Tumor - An abnormal growth that is not cancer and does not spread to other parts of the body.

Bilateral - Pertains to both sides of the body. For example, bilateral breast cancer would be on both sides of the body, or in both breasts.

Biopsy - The removal of a small piece of tissue, cells, or a small tumor for microscopic examination to determine if diseased cells are present. A biopsy is the most important procedure in diagnosing cancer.

Blood Count - A test to measure the number of red blood cells (RBCs), white blood cells (WBCs), platelets and blood chemistries from a blood sample.

Breast Cancer - Breast cells that are abnormal with uncontrolled growth. If not removed from the body, breast cancer may leave the breast, go to other vital organs in the body, continue to grow and become life threatening.

Breast Implants - A round or teardrop shaped sac inserted into the body to restore the shape of the breast. May be filled with saline water or synthetic material.

Breast Self-Exam (BSE) - A procedure practiced by a woman to examine the breast to detect any changes or suspicious lumps. Exams should be practiced monthly at the end of the period, or seven days after the start of the period; or for non-menstruating women, at the same time each month.

C

Calcifications - Small calcium deposits in breast tissue seen on a mammogram. The smallest object detected on mammography. Deposits are the result of cell death. Occurs with benign and malignant changes. Not related to dietary calcium intake.

Caffeine - A chemical in coffee, teas and other products that acts as a stimulate to the body.

Cancer - A general term used to describe more than 100 different uncontrolled growths of abnormal cells in the body. Cancer cells have the ability to continue to grow, invade and destroy surrounding tissue, leave the original site and travel via lymph or blood systems to other parts of the body where they can set up new cancerous tumors and become life threatening.

Cancer Cell - A cell that divides and reproduces abnormally with uncontrolled growth. This cell can break away and travel to other parts of the body and set up in another site, referred to as metastasis.

Clavicle - The collarbone.

Carcinogen - Any substance that initiates or promotes the development of cancer. For example, asbestos is a proven carcinogen.

Cell - The basic structural unit of all life. All living matter is composed of cells.

Cellulitis - Infection occurring in soft tissues. The surgical arm has an increased risk for cellulitis because of the removal of lymph nodes during breast cancer surgery. Pain, swelling and warmth occur in the area.

Colostrum - Fluid produced in the breasts during pregnancy and before the milk comes in.

Cooper's Ligaments - Small, flexible bands of tissue that pass from the chest muscle between the lobes of the breasts and provide shape and support.

Core Biopsy - Removal of a piece of a lump or calcifications with a large coring needle. The core tissue samples are sent to the lab to see if they are benign or malignant.

Costochondritis - Inflammation of the cartilage between the ribs that causes pain and tenderness that may radiate to the breast.

Cyclic Pain - Pain that changes in degree of intensity during a monthly hormonal cycle, increasing before menstruation and diminishing after menstruation.

Cyst - An abnormal sac-like structure that contains liquid or semi-solid material; is usually benign. Lumps in the breast are often found to be harmless cysts.

Cytology - Study of cells under a microscope that have been sloughed off, or scraped off organs to examine for signs of cancer.

Cytotoxic - Drugs that can cause the death of cancer cells. Usually refers to drugs used in chemotherapy treatments.

D

Detection - The discovery of an abnormality in an asymptomatic or symptomatic person.

Diagnosis - The process of identifying a disease by its characteristic signs, symptoms and laboratory findings. With cancer, the earlier the diagnosis is made, the better the chance for cure.

Dimpling - The pulling in of the skin on the surface of the breast, areola, or nipple.

Ductal Papillomas - Small, non-cancerous, finger-like growths in the mammary ducts that may cause a bloody nipple discharge. Commonly found in women 45 to 50 years of age.

Ductography - The insertion of a small plastic cannula into a milk duct of the breast through the nipple. The duct is injected with a dye by a radiologist. The duct can then be visualized by a radiologist using mammography to detect unusual filling of the dye in the duct, or seen by a surgeon during surgery.

E

Eczema - Irritation of the skin or nipple of a breast that may appear as redness, a rash, scaliness, or crusty areas, alone or in combination.

Edema - Excess fluid in the body or a body part described as swollen or puffy.

Endocrine Manipulation - The use of hormonal medications to treat breast problems.

Estrogen - A female hormone secreted by the ovaries which is essential for menstruation, reproduction and the development of secondary sex characteristics, such as breasts. Some patients with breast cancer are given drugs to suppress the production of estrogen in their bodies.

Estrogen Replacement Therapy (ERT) - Medication given to replace or supplement normal levels of estrogen in women.

Estrogen Receptor Assay (ERA) - A test that is done on cancerous tissue to see if a breast cancer is hormone-dependent and can be treated with hormonal therapy. The test will reveal if your cancer is estrogen receptor positive or negative.

Exaggerated Hormonal Response - Increased lumpiness or pain in the breasts that varies with monthly hormonal cycle. May cause mild to severe pain. Also may make breast self-exam difficult, due to an increased degree of lumpiness.

Excisional Biopsy - Surgical removal of a lump or suspicious tissue by cutting the skin and removing the lump or suspicious tissue.

F

Familial Cancer - One occurring in families more frequently than would be expected by chance.

Fat Necrosis Tumor - Destruction of fat cells in the breast due to trauma or injury that can cause a hard noncancerous lump.

Fibroadenoma - A noncancerous, solid tumor most commonly found in younger women.

Fibrocystic Breast Changes or Condition - A non-cancerous breast condition in which multiple cysts or lumpy areas develop in one or both breasts. It can be accompanied by discomfort or pain that fluctuates with the menstrual cycle.

Fine Needle Aspiration (FNA) - Procedure to remove cells or fluid from tissues using a needle with an empty syringe. Cells or breast fluid are extracted by pulling back on the plunger and are then analyzed by a pathologist.

Frozen Section - A technique in which a part of the biopsy tissue is frozen immediately, and a thin slice is then mounted on a microscope slide, enabling a pathologist to analyze it in just a few minutes for a diagnosis.

G

Galactocele - A clogged milk duct forming a cyst of milk that occurs during lactation (breast milk production).

Galactography - The insertion of a small, plastic cannula into a duct of the breast through the nipple. The duct is injected with a dye by a radiologist. The duct can then be visualized by a radiologist or seen by a surgeon during surgery.

Galactorrhea - A spontaneous discharge of breast milk not associated with breast-feeding.

Genes - Located in the nucleus of the cell, genes contain hereditary information that is transferred from cell to cell.

Genetic - Refers to the inherited pattern located in genes for certain characteristics.

H

Hematoma - A collection of blood that can form in a wound after surgery, an aspiration, or from an injury.

Herpes Zoster - A virus that causes shingles, a condition of small blisters on the skin, that causes pain.

Hormonal Therapy - Treatment of breast problems by alteration of the hormonal balance.

Hormone - Secreted by various organs in the body, hormones help regulate growth, metabolism and reproduction. Some hormones are used as treatment following surgery for breast, ovarian and prostate cancers.

Hormone Receptor Assay - A diagnostic test to determine whether a breast cancer's growth is influenced by hormones by having estrogen or progesterone receptors in its cells.

Hot Flashes - A sensation of heat and flushing that occurs suddenly. May be associated with menopause or some medications.

Hyperplasia - An abnormal, excessive growth of cells that is benign.

Hypothyroidism - Condition of low thyroid hormones in body causing low metabolic rate, fatigue, cold intolerance and breast pain.

I

Immune System - Complex system by which the body protects itself from outside invaders that are harmful to it.

Incisional Biopsy - A surgical incision made through the skin to remove a portion of a suspected lump or suspicious tissue.

Inflammation - Reaction of tissue to various conditions that may result in pain, redness, swelling, or warmth of tissues in the area.

Informed Consent - Process of explanation to the patient of all risks and complications of a procedure or treatment before it is done. Most informed consents are written and signed by the patient or a legal representative.

Intraductal - Residing within the duct of the breast. Intraductal disease may be benign or malignant.

Invasive Cancer - Cancer that has spread outside its site of origin and is growing into the surrounding tissues.

In Situ - In place, localized and confined to one area. A very early stage of cancer found inside the duct or lobule that has not grown through cell wall of where it began.

Infiltrating Ductal Cell Carcinoma - A cancer that begins in the mammary duct and has spread through the cell wall where it began to areas outside the duct.

Intravenous (IV) - Method of giving medications or nutrition into a vein after insertion of a needle.

Inverted Nipple - The turning inward of the nipple. Usually a congenital condition; but, if it occurs where it has not previously existed, it can be a sign of breast cancer or benign breast disease.

L

Lactation - Process of producing milk from the breasts.

Lactational Mastitis - Inflammation of breast glands during breast-feeding causing tenderness, pain and fever.

Lactiferous Sinus - Enlarged area of a milk duct, located close to the nipple, that acts as a reservoir for breast milk before breastfeeding.

Lesion - An area of tissue in normal tissues that has changed and that's presence can be distinguished by palpation or imaging studies. May be benign or malignant.

Lobular - Pertaining to the part of the breast that is furthest from the nipple, the end portion of the lobes where milk is produced.

Lump - Any kind of abnormal mass in the breast or elsewhere in the body. May be malignant or benign.

Lumpectomy - A surgical procedure in which only the cancerous tumor and an area of surrounding tissue is removed. Usually the surgeon will remove some of the underarm lymph nodes at the same time. This procedure is also referred to as a tylectomy.

Lymphatic Vessels - Vessels that remove cellular waste and infection from the body by filtering through lymph nodes and eventually emptying into the vascular (blood) system.

Lymph - A clear fluid that circulates throughout the body in the lymphatic system; contains white blood cells and antibodies.

Lymph Gland - Also called a lymph node. These are round-bodied tissues in the lymphatic system that vary in size from a pinhead to an olive and may appear alone or in groups. The principal ones are in the neck, underarm and groin. These glands produce lymphocytes and monocytes (white blood cells which fight foreign substances) and serve as filters to prevent bacteria from entering the bloodstream. They filter out cancer cells but also serve as a site for metastatic disease. The major ones serving the breast are in the armpit. Some are located above and below the collarbone and some in between the ribs near the breastbone. There are three levels of lymph nodes in the underarm area of the breast and another one around the breastbone. The number of nodes varies from person to person. Lymph nodes are usually sampled during surgery to determine if the cancer has spread outside of the breast area.

Lymphedema - A swelling in the arm caused by excess fluid that collects after the lymph nodes have been removed by surgery or affected by radiation treatments.

M

Macrocyst - A cyst that is large and can usually be felt with the fingers.

Magnification View - Special enlarged views used in mammography to magnify an area for a more detailed examination of a suspicious finding.

Malignant Tumor - A mass of cancer cells. These cells have uncontrolled growth and will invade surrounding tissues and spread to distant sites of the body, setting up new cancer sites which are potentially life threatening.

Mammary Duct Ectasia - A non-cancerous breast disease most often found in women right before and during menopause. The ducts in or beneath the nipple become clogged with cellular and fatty debris. The duct may have a whitish gray to greenish discharge. The area may become inflamed and cause pain or can develop into an infection that can cause an abscess.

Mammary Dysplasia - An alteration in size or shape of breast glands that is benign.

Mammary Glands - The breast glands that produce and carry milk by way of the mammary ducts to the nipples during pregnancy and breast- feeding.

Mammary Ridge or Inframammary Ridge - A ridge of firm tissue located at the base of the breasts along the underwire area of a bra.

Mammogram - An x-ray of the breast that can detect tumors before they can be felt. A baseline mammogram is performed on healthy breasts usually at the age of 35 to establish a basis for later comparison

Mammotest® - Biopsy performed under mammography while breast is compressed; the lesion is viewed by a physician. Sample of lesion is removed using a large core needle and is then sent to a lab to determine if it is benign or malignant. Also known as stereotactic biopsy.

Margins - The area of tissue surrounding a tumor when it is removed by surgery. Clear margins mean no cancer was seen at the edges of biopsy specimen. Dirty margins or unclear margins mean that cancer cells were still seen under the microscope.

Mastalgia - Pain occurring in the breast.

Mastectomy - Surgical removal of the entire breast and some of the surrounding tissue. Types of mastectomies:

> **Modified Radical Mastectomy** - The most common type of mastectomy. Breast skin, nipple, areola and underarm lymph nodes are removed. The chest muscles are saved.

> **Prophylactic Mastectomy** - A procedure sometimes recommended for patients at a very high risk for developing cancer to remove breasts as a prevention measure. Women after breast cancer surgery may have prophylactic mastectomy to remove opposite breast for bilateral reconstruction or reduce risk for future cancer in breast.

> **Subcutaneous mastectomy** - Performed before cancer is detected, removes the breast tissue but leaves the outer skin, areola and nipple intact. (This is not suitable with a diagnosis of cancer.)

> **Radical Mastectomy** (Halsted Radical) - The surgical removal of the breast, breast skin, nipple, areola, chest muscles and underarm lymph nodes.

> **Segmental Mastectomy** (Partial Mastectomy/Lumpectomy) - A surgical procedure in which only a portion of the breast is removed, including the cancer and the surrounding margin of healthy breast tissue.

Mastitis - Infection occurring in the breast. Pain, tenderness, swelling, redness and warmth may be observed. Usually related to infection and will respond to antibiotic treatment.

Menopause - The time in a woman's life when the menstrual cycle ends because the ovaries produce lower levels of hormones; usually occurs between the age of 45 and 55.

Metastasis - The spread of cancer from one part of the body to another through the lymphatic system or the bloodstream. The cells in the new cancer location are the same type as those in the original site.

Microcalcifications - Particles observed on a mammogram that are found in the breast tissue appearing as small spots on the picture. Usually occur from calcium deposits caused by death of breast cells; may be benign or malignant. When clustered in one area, may need to be checked more closely for a malignant change in the breast.

Microcyst - A cyst that is too small to be felt but may be observed on a mammogram or ultrasound screening.

Micrometastasis - Undetectable spread of cancer outside the breast that is not seen on routine screening tests. Metastasis is too limited to have created enough mass to be observed.

Mondor's Syndrome - An inflamed vein in the breast caused by a clot, that may occur after trauma, muscular strain, radiation therapy, or surgical procedures. May also be called "breast phlebitis" or "superficial periphlebitis".

Montgomery's Glands - Small oil glands that lubricate the nipple of the breast during lactation.

Multicentric - Having more than one origin or place of growth in the breast. These areas may or may not be related to each other.

Musculoskeletal Pain - Breast pain that is caused by a pinched nerve in the back, a back injury, scoliosis, arthritis, or osteoporosis.

MRI (magnetic resonance imaging) - Imaging test of internal body parts using large magnets to produce a series of pictures for diagnosis of disease.

N

Needle Biopsy - Removal of a sample of tissue from the breast using a large-coring needle.

Necrosis - Death of a tissue.

Neoplasm - Any abnormal growth. Neoplasms may be benign or malignant, but the term is commonly used to describe a cancer.

Nipple - The darker, protruding portion of the breast that has openings that allow breast milk to be expelled during breastfeeding.

Nodularity - Increased density of breast tissue, most often due to hormonal changes in the breast, which cause the breast to feel lumpy. This finding is called normal nodularity, and usually occurs in both breasts.

Nodule - A small, solid mass.

Noncyclic Pain - Breast pain that does not change with the monthly hormonal cycle. May be occasional or chronic.

Normal Nodularity - The normal feeling of lumpiness, with no firm, obvious, single, hard lump; caused by influence of female hormones on breast tissue. Lumpiness will vary according to the monthly hormonal cycle and be most noticeable before a menstrual period.

O

Oncogene - Certain portions of cellular DNA. Genes that, when inappropriately activated, contribute to the malignant transformation of a cell.

One-Step Procedure - A procedure in which a surgical biopsy is performed under general anesthesia. If cancer is found, a mastectomy or lumpectomy is done immediately as part of the same operation. This is rarely done today.

Oophorectomy - The surgical removal of the ovaries, sometimes performed as a part of hormone therapy.

Orange Peel Skin - Skin looks dimpled like the peel of an orange. The pitted appearance is caused from inflammation and edema of the breast caused by benign or cancerous diseases.

Osteoporosis - A softening of bones that occurs with age, calcium loss and hormone depletion.

P

Palliative Treatment - Therapy that relieves symptoms, such as pain or pressure, but does not alter the development of the disease. Its primary purpose is to improve the quality of life.

Palpation - A procedure using the hands to examine organs such as the breast. A palpable mass is one you can feel with your hands.

Papilloma - A small benign growth in the breast ducts identified as having a mushroom like appearance (stalk).

Pathology - The study of disease through the microscopic examination of body tissues. Any tumor suspected of being cancerous must be diagnosed by pathological examination.

Pathologist - A physician with special training in diagnosing diseases from samples of tissue.

Pectoralis Muscles - Muscular tissues that are under the breasts; attached to the front of the chest wall and extending to the upper arms. They are divided into the pectoralis major and the pectoralis minor muscles.

Perimenopausal - Several years before and the period right after the onset of menopause.

Permanent Section - A technique in which a thin slice of biopsy tissue is mounted on a slide to be examined under a microscope by a pathologist in order to establish a diagnosis.

Pharmacological Discharge - Breast discharge caused by medications and comes from both breasts. Not caused by normal changes in hormonal levels.

Phlebitis - Inflammation of a vein causing pain.

Phyllodes Tumor - Tumor found in the breast that is usually benign, but can occasionally be malignant.

Physiological Discharge - A cloudy, bilateral breast discharge that is caused by changes in monthly hormonal levels.

Precancerous - Abnormal cellular changes that are potentially capable of becoming cancer. These early lesions are very amenable to treatment and cure. Also called pre-malignant.

Premenstrual Syndrome (PMS) - A combination of emotional and physical changes occurring in an ovulating woman that peaks the week before the onset of the menstrual period.

Progesterone - Female hormone produced by the ovaries during a specific time in the menstrual cycle. Causes the uterus to prepare for pregnancy and the breasts to get ready to produce milk.

Prognosis - A prediction of the course of the disease—the future prospect for the patient. For example, most breast cancer patients who receive treatment early have a good prognosis.

Prolactin - The female hormone that stimulates the development of the breast and later is essential for starting and continuing milk production.

R

Radiologist - A physician who specializes in diagnoses of diseases by the use of x-rays or other imaging studies such as magnetic resonance imaging (MRI).

Recurrence - Reappearance of cancer after a period of remission.

Remission - Complete or partial disappearance of the signs and symptoms of disease in response to treatment. The period when a disease is under control. A remission, however, is not necessarily a cure.

Retraction - Process of skin pulling in toward breast tissue. Often referred to as dimpling.

Risk Factors - Anything that increases an individual's chance of getting a disease. Some of the most common risk factors for breast disease are a first or second degree relative with breast cancer on mother's or father's side diagnosed at an early age, ovarian cancer in the family at any age, early menstruation, late menopause, first child after 30 or no children.

Risk Reduction - Techniques used to reduce chances of getting a certain cancer. For example, reducing alcohol consumption may reduce risk.

S

Sclerosing Adenosis - A condition of increased thickness or hardness in the area of the milk producing units, the acini. This condition is benign.

Screening Mammogram - A two-view mammogram on each breast used to screen a woman for breast cancer when no known abnormality exists in the breasts.

Spiculated - Appearing on mammography as small projections into surrounding tissues from a mass, forming a star-burst appearance.

Stellate - Appearing on mammography as a star-shape because of the irregular growth of cells into surrounding tissue. May be associated with a malignancy or some benign conditions.

Stereotactic Needle Biopsy - Biopsy done while breast is compressed under mammography. A series of pictures locate the lesion, and a radiologist enters information into a computer. The computer calculates information and positions a needle to sample the lesion. A needle is inserted into the lump, and pieces of tissue are removed and sent to a lab for analysis. May be referred to as Mammotest® or core needle biopsy.

Supraclavicular Nodes - The nodes located above the collarbone in the area of the neck.

T

Tamoxifen - An anti-estrogen drug that may be given to women with estrogen receptive tumors to block estrogen from entering the breast tissues. May produce menopause-like symptoms, including hot flashes and vaginal dryness. Currently being used with high-risk women in clinical trials to prevent breast cancer, and with women who have had breast cancer to prevent recurrence.

Tissue - A collection of similar cells. There are four basic types of tissues in the body: epithelial, connective, muscle, and nerve.

Trauma - Injury to the breast.

Tumor - An abnormal collection of tissues in an area. May be also called a lesion or mass. Tumors may be either benign or malignant.

Two-Step Procedure - When surgical biopsy and breast surgery are performed in two separate surgeries.

U

Ultrasound Examination - The use of high frequency sound waves to locate a tumor inside the body. Helps determine if a breast lump is solid tissue or filled with fluids.

Ultrasound Guided Biopsy or Localization - The use of ultrasound to guide a biopsy needle to obtain a sample of tissue for biopsy or to place localization wires prior to surgery. Physician can view the movement of the needle in real-time and pictures can be taken to verify placement or removal of tissues.

Unilateral - Pertains to one breast. Located on one side of the body.

REFERENCES

Ajmera P.R., Larbi A.B., Gebhardt G., et al., *PDR Guide to Drug Interactions, Side Effects, Indications.* Montvale, NJ: Medical Economics Company, Inc. 2002.

Bennett B.B., Steinbach B.G, Hardt N.S., and Haigh L.S., *Breast Disease for Clinicians,* New York, NY: McGraw Hill, 2001

Bland K.I. and Copeland III E.M., *The Breast.* Philadelphia, PA: W. B. Saunders Company, 1991.

Bohmert H.H. and Leis Jr. P.H., *Breast Cancer.* New York, NY: Thieme Medical, 1989.

Food and Drug Administration Medwatch, FDA Medical Bulletin, *Botanical Dietary Supplement Adverse Effects*, 994. 24 (No2): 3, Drugdex (R) Editorial Staff.

Dixon J.M. and Morrow M., *Breast Disease: A Problem-Based Approach.* New York: W.B. Saunders, 1999

Spratt J.S. and Donegan W.L., *Cancer of the Breast.* Philadelphia, PA: W.B. Saunders Company, l995.

Lippman M.E., Morrow M., Hellman S., and Harris J.R., *Diseases of the Breast.* Philadelphia, PA: Lippincott-Raven, 1996.

Hudson, Tori, *Women's Encyclopedia of Natural Medicine.* Los Angeles, CA: Keats Publishing, 1999

Hughes L.E., Mansel R.E., and Webster D.J.T., *Benign Disorders and Diseases of the Breast.* Philadelphia, PA: W.B. Saunders, 2000

Hunt K.K., Robb G.L, Strom E.A., and Ueno N.T. *Breast Cancer* (M.D. Anderson Cancer Series). New York, NY: Springer-Verlag, 2001

Marchant D.J., *Contemporary Management of Breast Diseases: Benign Disease.* Philadelphia, PA: W. B. Saunders, 1994.

Physicians Desk Reference, Breast Cancer Disease Management, Montvale, NJ: Medical Economics Company, Inc. 2002

Pazdur R., Coia L.R., Hoskins W.J., and Wagman L.D., *Cancer Management: A Multidisciplinary Approach.* Melville, NY: PRR, 2002

PDR for Herbal Medicines, Montvale, NJ: Medical Economics Company, Inc. 1998

Silva O.E. and Zurrida S., *Breast Cancer: A Practical Guide*, New York, NY: Elsevier Science Ltd., 2000

INDEX

O

oil glands 57
oral contraceptive 90, 98
orange peel skin 26, 111
osteoporosis 35, 83, 87
ovarian cancer 59, 96, 97, 98
ovarian glands 42
ovaries 98

P

papilloma 53
pathologist 72, 79, 80
pathology report 78, 80
PDR® 117, 129
pectoralis 14
percutaneous 73
periductal mastitis 51
perimenopausal 40
pesticides 89
phyllodes tumor (phylloides) 50
Physician's Desk Reference 117
pituitary gland 42
plasma cell mastitis 51
PMS 36
PMS symptoms 44
postmenopausal 86
pregnancy 17, 21
Premarin 84, 85, 86, 87
pre-menopausal 34, 37, 94
pre-menstrual symptoms 36
pre-menstrual syndrome 33
Prempro 84, 85, 86
progesterone 15, 34, 39, 40,
    43, 85, 86
progesterone supplementation 39
progestin 82, 85
prolactin 39, 41, 42, 43

Provera 84, 85, 86
pseudoephedrine 35
psychiatric medications 43
puberty 18

R

radiation 30
radiation therapy 55, 56
radiographic dye 53
reconstructive surgery 113

S

scar tissue 64
sclerosing adenosis 56
scoliosis 35
screening mammogram 61, 63
seroma 71
sexual stimulation 30, 41, 110
shingles 57
skin changes 26
skin dimpling 27
skin retraction 52
spot compression 61, 63
stereotactic biopsy 73
stereotactic core needle biopsy 61
steroid 35, 38
stroma 50
superficial periphlebitis 56
surgical biopsy 69, 75, 76

T

Tamoxifen 98
thyroid 40, 42
thyroid function 40
thyroid gland 34, 42
Tietze's syndrome 35
tissue structures 63
transdermal 87
trauma 56
tumor 42

U

ultrasound 36, 45, 47, 48, 61,
   66, 67, 73, 76, 98
unilateral 44
urination 83
uterine cancer 84
uterus 31

V

vacuum assisted core biopsy 69, 74
vaginal dryness 83
vaginal ring 88
vein changes 27
vitamin 32, 38

W

wire localization 71

X

x-ray 61, 76

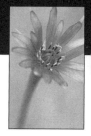

Breast Self-Exam *Calendar*

Tear out this calendar and place it where it will serve as a reminder to perform your *monthly* breast self-exam. Note the date of your exam in the space provided, and the date of your mammogram. After you complete your exam each month, congratulate yourself for taking an active part in your breast health!

January	February	March	April
May	June	July	August
September	October	November	December

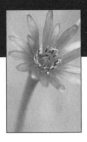

Breast Self-Exam *Reminders*

Successful breast care is a combination of three components – breast self-exam, clinical exam by a physician and mammography on the recommended schedule. Each one can identify breast abnormalities that the other may miss.

The best time to perform your monthly exam:

■ **Pre-menopausal women –**
the conclusion of your monthly period.

■ **Menopausal or pregnant women –**
select a day each month that is easy for your to remember.

■ **Women on hormonal medications –**
if you cycle off your medication for several days each month–
perform your exam on the day your resume your medication.

■ **Breastfeeding women –**
examine your breasts after you have emptied the breast of
milk; sometimes this may require that you examine only one
breast at a time because all the milk may not be expressed
completely from both breasts.

■ **Check your breasts <u>only once a month</u> unless you identify a
problem that needs to be monitored.**

■ **Have a clinical exam by a physician once a year.**

■ **Have your mammogram on the recommended basis.**

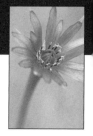

Breast Self-Exam *Record*

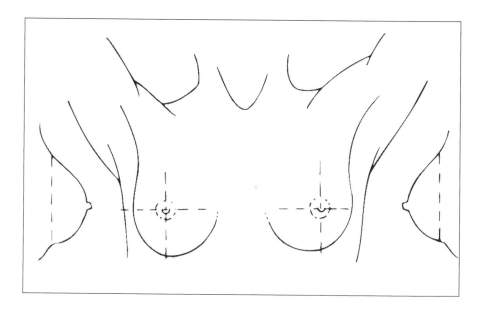

Date of Exam: _____ **Time in Cycle:** _____

Mark areas where you find changes during your breast exam. Identify changes and mark accordingly.

See chart on back of this page for description of symptoms.

Change	Right Breast	Left Breast
Thickening	☐	☐
Lump	☐	☐
Soft	☐	☐
Firm	☐	☐
Moveable	☐	☐
Non-Moveable	☐	☐
Bulge	☐	☐
Color Change	☐	☐
Dimpling	☐	☐
Vein Pattern Change	☐	☐
Nipple/Areola	☐	☐
Orange Peel Skin	☐	☐
Nipple Discharge	☐	☐
Change Size/Shape	☐	☐
Bump/Sore/Rash	☐	☐
Lymph Node	☐	☐

Mark the approximate size of the lump or lymph node that you discovered. Use this record when you go to your healthcare provider or recheck the area next month to see if the area becomes smaller or larger.

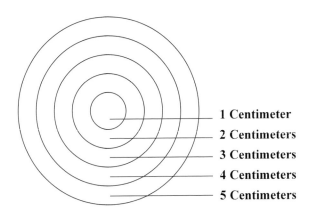

1 Centimeter
2 Centimeters
3 Centimeters
4 Centimeters
5 Centimeters

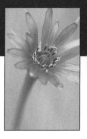

Physician's *Worksheet*

If you need a biopsy of a suspicious area, ask your healthcare provider to draw where the area is found in your breast. If you are to have an incisional or excisional biopsy, ask you healthcare provider to draw where and how the scar will look.

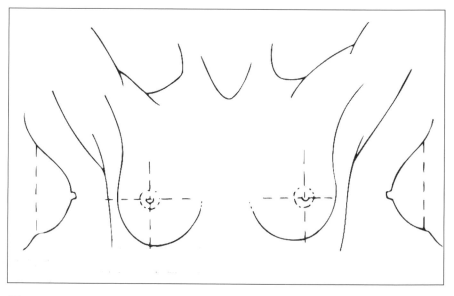

Have your healthcare provider draw the size of your lump.

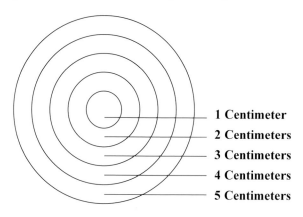

1 Centimeter
2 Centimeters
3 Centimeters
4 Centimeters
5 Centimeters

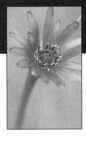

Biopsy *Instructions*

Patient: _____

Healthcare Provider: _____

Date: _____ Time: _____

Type of biopsy: _____

Type of anesthesia: ☐ local   ☐ general

Special instructions **before** biopsy: _____

_____

_____

_____

Special instructions **after** biopsy: _____

_____

_____

_____

Call Healthcare Provider when:

- Temperature is over _____.

- Pain uncontrolled with prescribed medications.

- Signs of new bleeding that doesn't stop in a few minutes with a pressure bandage.

- Sudden pain and swelling at the biopsy site.

- Yellow or greenish drainage from incisional scar area several days after biopsy.

- Foul-smelling discharge on dressing.

Other: _____

Biopsy report will be available: _____

For questions or assistance call: _____

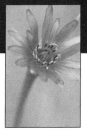

Breast Pain *Description*

Name: _____ Age: _____

Birth Control Pills:	☐ yes	☐ no
Menopausal:	☐ yes	☐ no
Estrogen Replacement:	☐ yes	☐ no

Kind of Pain:
Describe your pain by checking the following descriptive terms:
- ☐ Tender to touch _____
- ☐ Dull, Aching _____
- ☐ Throbbing _____
- ☐ Burning sensation _____
- ☐ Sharp, stabbing _____
- ☐ Other _____

Where does it hurt?
Mark on this diagram the area where you feel the pain. If the pain radiates from the breast, draw an arrow in the direction it radiates.

☐ One breast

☐ Both breasts

☐ Pain localized

☐ Pain generalized

☐ Near surface of breast

☐ Pain deep in breast

161

How and when did the pain begin?

Sudden onset of pain?	☐ yes	☐ no
Is it increasing?	☐ yes	☐ no
How long have you had pain?	_____	

When is it painful?

At rest	☐ yes	☐ no
When walking or exercising	☐ yes	☐ no
When taking a deep breath or stretching	☐ yes	☐ no
Only when touched or with movement	☐ yes	☐ no
Does it keep you from going to sleep	☐ yes	☐ no
Does it awaken you from sleep	☐ yes	☐ no

What relieves the pain?

Aspirin/Tylenol®/Ibuprofen	☐ yes	☐ no
Wearing a bra	☐ yes	☐ no
No activity	☐ yes	☐ no
Heat	☐ yes	☐ no
Cold	☐ yes	☐ no
Other	_____	

Do you drink or take?

Coffee	☐ yes	☐ no
Soft Drinks containing caffeine	☐ yes	☐ no
Herbal products	☐ yes	☐ no
Over-the-counter pain/diet/energy pills	☐ yes	☐ no
Supplemental estrogen/birth control pills	☐ yes	☐ no
Medications: List	_____	

_____

_____

Fill in this information for your healthcare provider. This will be helpful in gathering clues, patterns and connections which can help identify the probable cause of your breast pain.

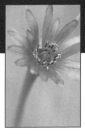

Breast Pain *Assessment Chart*

Name: _____ Age: _____

Date Started: _____ Date Completed: _____

Record your daily amount of breast pain on this chart. Careful recording of the pain will enable your healthcare provider to determine possible causes.

Mark the following information on your calendar:

- Day you begin your menstrual period - MP1 (menstrual period day 1).

- Day your menstrual period ends - MPS (menstrual period stopped).

- If you are menopausal, mark MX at the beginning of the chart.

- Chart pain on a scale, rating pain in a range from 0 (no pain) to 10 (severe pain).

- Chart the area in the breast where the pain occurs; see breast diagram below for numbers. The breast is divided into four quadrants. You may select one or multiple areas of the breasts. Example: LB 1, 3, 4.

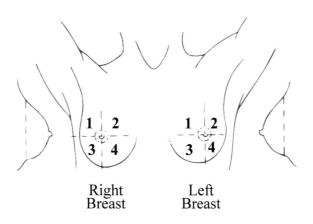

Right Breast   Left Breast

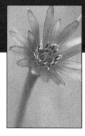

Breast Pain *Assessment Chart*

- Note time of day pain is experienced:
  AM (midnight to noon)
  PM (noon to midnight)
  AD (all day)

- On each day pain is experienced, record unusual physical activities performed.

- Note any unusual dietary changes on days pain is experienced (more or less consumption of caffeine, etc.).

- Note any medication usage (cold pills, herbal products, prescription medications. etc.).

Example of one day's charting:
Saturday, January 1
MP1 (menstrual period day 1)
Pain #6
LB3 (left breast, area 3)
AD (all day)
Tennis
1 Coffee, 2 Cokes, Herbal Tea, Cold Pills X2

Charting Abbreviations:

AD	All Day
AM	Midnight to Noon
LB	Left Breast
MP1	Menstrual Period Day 1
MPS	Menstrual Period Stopped
MX	Menopausal
PM	Noon to Midnight
RB	Right Breast

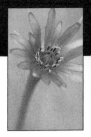

Breast Pain *Assessment Calendar*

	Week 1	Week 2
Sunday		
Monday		
Tuesday		
Wednesday		
Thursday		
Friday		
Saturday		

Breast Pain *Assessment Calendar*

	Week 3	Week 4
Sunday		
Monday		
Tuesday		
Wednesday		
Thursday		
Friday		
Saturday		

EduCare *Worksheet*

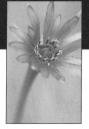

Breast Discharge *Assessment*

Name: _____ Age: _____

Date Started: _____ Date Completed: _____

Record on your calendar the dates you have a breast(s) discharge. Careful recording of the discharge and possible promoters will help your healthcare provider evaluate the cause.

Mark the following information on your calendar:

- Day you begin your menstrual period - MP1
  (menstrual period day 1).

- Day your menstrual period ends - MPS
  (menstrual period stopped).

- If you are menopausal, mark MX at the beginning of the chart.

- Chart amount of discharge - rating amount from:

  0 = None
  1 = Few drops
  2 = Small amount found in bra
  3 = Large amount found in bra

- Note the breast that has the discharge -
  Left Breast (LB), Right Breast (RB).

- Look at your nipple carefully to see if the discharge is from one area of the nipple. Look at the chart below and the numbers identifying the areas. Select the number(s) of the area(s) of the nipple which produce the discharge.

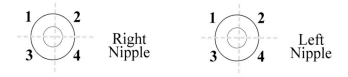

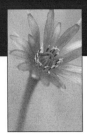

Breast Discharge *Assessment*

- Note the color of the discharge: C (clear), B (bloody red), P (pinkish), G (gray), B (brown), Y (yellow), M (milky).

- Note time of day the discharge is experienced: AM (midnight to noon), PM (noon to midnight), AD (all day).

- On each day a discharge is experienced, record unusual physical activities performed.

- Note any unusual dietary changes on days a discharge is experienced (more or less consumption of caffeine, etc.).

- Note any medication usage (cold pills, herbal products, prescription medications. etc.).

Example of one day's charting:
Saturday, January 1
MP1 (menstrual period day 1)
LB4 (left breast, area 4)
2 (small amount in bra)
M (milky)
AD (all day)
Tennis
1 Coffee, 2 Cokes, Herbal Tea, Cold Pills X2

Charting Abbreviations:

AD	All Day
AM	Midnight to Noon
LB	Left Breast
MP1	Menstrual Period Day 1
MPS	Menstrual Period Stopped
MX	Menopausal
PM	Noon to Midnight
RB	Right Breast

EduCare *Worksheet*

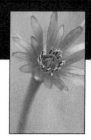

Breast Discharge *Assessment Calendar*

	Week 1	Week 2
Sunday		
Monday		
Tuesday		
Wednesday		
Thursday		
Friday		
Saturday		

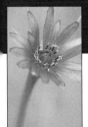

EduCare *Worksheet*

Breast Discharge *Assessment Calendar*

	Week 3	Week 4
Sunday		
Monday		
Tuesday		
Wednesday		
Thursday		
Friday		
Saturday		

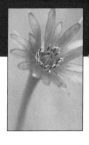

Drugs That I Take

List any medications that have been prescribed by a healthcare provider, over-the-counter medications, and herbal products that you take either occasionally or on a regular basis.

Prescription Drugs: _____

_____

_____

_____

_____

_____

Over-the-Counter Drugs: _____

_____

_____

_____

_____

_____

Herbal Products: _____

_____

_____

_____

_____

_____

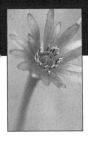

EduCare *Worksheet*

Patient Appointment *Worksheet*

What I Need To Ask or Tell My Healthcare Team

Next Scheduled Appointment:

Healthcare Provider: _____

Place: _____ Date: _____ Time: _____

Questions To Ask Physician: _____

_____

_____

_____

_____

Questions To Ask Nurse: _____

_____

_____

_____

Remember To Tell Physician/Nurse: _____

_____

_____

_____

_____

It is helpful to write down questions for your nurse or physician prior to your visit and have them answered. It is also helpful to keep a list of items which need to be relayed to your healthcare team.

EduCare *Worksheet*

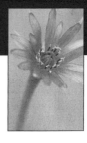

Patient Appointment *Worksheet*

What I Need To Ask or Tell My Healthcare Team

Next Scheduled Appointment:

Healthcare Provider: _____

Place: _____ Date: _____ Time: _____

Questions To Ask Physician: _____
_____
_____
_____
_____

Questions To Ask Nurse: _____
_____
_____
_____
_____

Remember To Tell Physician/Nurse: _____
_____
_____
_____
_____

It is helpful to write down questions for your nurse or physician prior to your visit and have them answered. It is also helpful to keep a list of items which need to be relayed to your healthcare team.

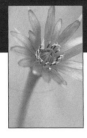

EduCare *Worksheet*

Patient Appointment *Worksheet*
What I Need To Ask or Tell My Healthcare Team

Next Scheduled Appointment:

Healthcare Provider: _____

Place: _____ Date: _____ Time: _____

Questions To Ask Physician: _____

_____

_____

_____

Questions To Ask Nurse: _____

_____

_____

_____

Remember To Tell Physician/Nurse: _____

_____

_____

_____

It is helpful to write down questions for your nurse or physician prior to your visit and have them answered. It is also helpful to keep a list of items which need to be relayed to your healthcare team.